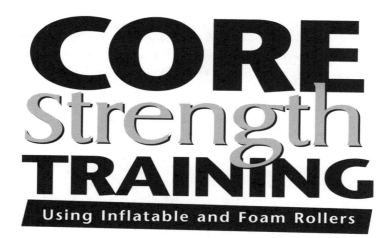

CORE Strength TRAINING
Using Inflatable and Foam Rollers

D1534116

© Caroline Corning Creager, 2006

Library of Congress Card Number: 94-90684
Creager, Caroline Corning
        Core Strength Training Using Inflatable and Foam Rollers
        Creager, Caroline Corning - 1st edition

FitNiche Publishing
Formerly known as Executive Physical Therapy, Inc.
P.O. Box 1319
Berthoud, CO 80513
(970) 532-2533
1-800-530-6878
email: Caroline@CarolineCreager.com

Printed in the United States of America

The author has made every effort to assure that the information in this book is accurate and current at the time of printing. The publisher and author take no responsibility for the use of the material in this book and cannot be held responsible for any typographical or other errors found. Please consult your physician before initiating this exercise program. The information in this book is not intended to replace medical advice.

ISBN: 0-9641153-6-0
Library of Congress Card Number: 94-90684

Cover Design by Kathy Tracy
Book Design by Kelly Keller and Kathy Tracy
Photographs by Jon Youngblut
Illustrations by Amy Brickey
Editing by Art Adams

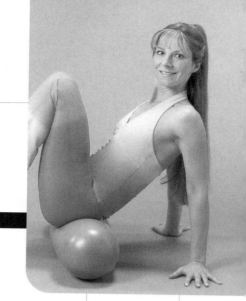

About the Author:
Caroline Corning Creager, P.T.

Caroline Corning Creager is an award-winning author and an internationally recognized speaker on fitness and physical therapy topics. Caroline received her degree in Physical Therapy from the University of Montana. She is the Owner and C.E.O. of FitNiche Publishing, the Berthoud Athletic Club, and Executive Physical Therapy, Inc. in Berthoud, Colorado, U.S.A., and author of seven books: *Bounce Back Into Shape After Baby, Therapeutic Exercises Using Foam Rollers, Therapeutic Exercises Using the Swiss Ball, Therapeutic Exercises Using Resistive Bands, Caroline Creager's Airobic Ball Strengthening Workout, Caroline Creager's Airobic Ball Stretching Workout,* and the most recent *Core Strength Training Using Inflatable and Foam Rollers.*

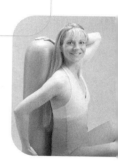

She has written or been featured in numerous national and international magazines: *Cooking Light, Fitness, Fit, Tennis, Yoga Journal, Massage Therapy Journal, WorldWideSpine, PhysioForum, Advance for PT's, Advance for OT's, Advance for Nurses, Idea Personal Trainer,* and *Baby Steps,* and has been a guest speaker for local television stations, and national programs: America's Talking: Alive and Wellness, and the Rehab Training Network.

Dedications

To my daughter, Alexis Eliana, who I was 3 months pregnant with during the photo shoot for this book. Alexis, your radiant spirit has been a welcome addition to the family.

To my boys, Michael and Christopher, whose energy and zest for life require me to stay in shape so that I can keep up with them.

To my husband Robert — I keep hoping, sweetheart, that you will learn to love exercise as much as I love you.

To the members and instructors of the Berthoud Athletic Club, and my clients from Executive Physical Therapy, Inc., I learn from you each and every day.

Preface

Life long health and fitness has been my aspiration for many years and will continue to be for the years to come. However, finding time to exercise daily continues to be a struggle for me, and my clients. That infamous TIME is one element in life that is limited and I never seem to be able to find more of it.

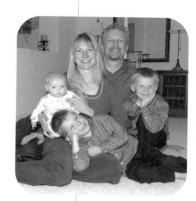

With the recent birth of my third child, finding time to exercise has become even more difficult. Fortunately I have become smarter about how I exercise, and the inflatable and foam rollers are not only essential to a time and energy-efficient exercise program, they are ideal for strengthening your core muscles.

I have learned that one does not always benefit more from longer or time-intensive workouts. Shorter workouts that continually challenge the body can be more effective than longer workouts that are repetitive in nature.

I hope you enjoy all of the inflatable and foam roller exercises and have fun strengthening YOUR CORE.

Caroline C. Creager, P.T.

In Memory Of:

Sue Annette Creager

May the road rise up to meet you,
May the wind be always at your back,
May the sun shine warm upon your face,
And the rains fall soft upon your fields,
And until we meet again,
May God hold you in the palm of His hand.

An Irish Blessing

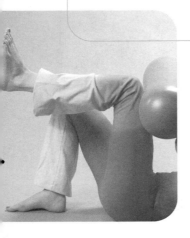

Contents

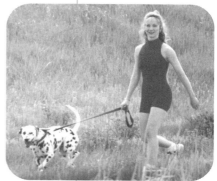

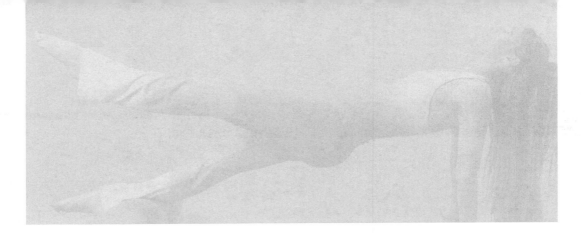

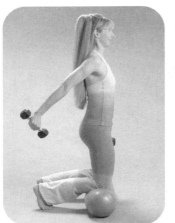

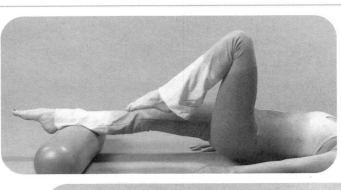

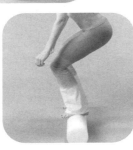

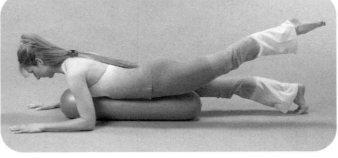

Introduction

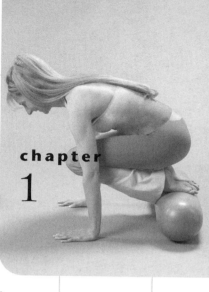

Do you realize your core muscles – the muscles of the abdomen, back, hips, and pelvic floor – affect how your entire body functions? Strong or weak core muscles determine if you will have poor or good posture, if you'll become injured or stay healthy, or if you will live with or without pain.

Your core is your body's infrastructure – and a strong, flexible muscular foundation is your best protection against injury. Core muscle strength is also necessary for proper posture, lifting, performing activities of daily living and any type of sport or exercise.

Core Strength Training Using Inflatable and Foam Rollers focuses on strengthening your core muscles. This book will also teach you how to make simple changes to your daily workout routine to improve your core strength and provide you with fun, time, and energy-efficient workouts. You will be able to work out at your own pace in the convenience of your own home or squeeze exercises in where and when your tight work schedule permits.

Whether you want to strengthen your arms (see illustration 1.1), tone your abdomen, or relieve tension in your lower back, you will find information to do so and learn balanced strengthening and stretching workouts. Each exercise page provides easy-to-read directions, illustrations, or photographs

> Strong or weak core muscles determine if you will have poor or good posture, if you'll become injured or stay healthy, or if you will live with or without pain.

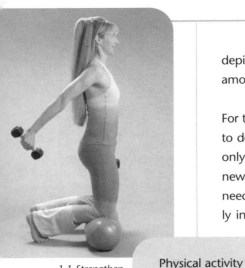

1.1 Strengthen Your Arms

depicting how to do the exercise, and mini-workouts that note the amount of time required to complete them.

For the majority of the population, it is very difficult to find a block of time to do a 30 – 60 minute workout. I have found that on some days I may only have a 10-minute block of time to squeeze in a workout. Good news: The Surgeon General's Report, 1996, states that, "physical activity need not be strenuous to achieve health benefits. People who are usually inactive can improve their health and well-being by becoming even moderately active on a regular basis. Greater health benefits can be achieved by increasing the amount [duration, frequency, or intensity] of physical activity."

> Physical activity can be accumulated through the day in shorter bouts of 10-minute durations.
> — *American College of Sports Medicine*

Research at the University of Pittsburgh School of Medicine found that exercising in 10-minute time increments, several times a day, could be just as beneficial as working out for 30 minutes once a day. The American College of Sports Medicine (Med Sci Sports Exerc., 1998) also reports "many health benefits from physical activity can be achieved at lower intensities of exercise, if frequency and duration of training are increased appropriately. In this regard, physical activity can be accumulated through the day in shorter bouts of 10-minute durations."

How To Use This Book
One Star to Five Star Rating System

Starting a new exercise program can be intimidating. For this reason, I have rated each exercise on a one to five star system. One star signifies the most basic exercise level, two stars – advanced beginner, three stars (see illustration 1.2) – intermediate, four stars – advanced, and five stars – expert. The star rating is located at the top of the page. If the exercise received one star, then you will know right away that it may be performed by a beginner, and a five star exercise means you may need to wait awhile before you perform it, or that this exercise is for you if you are already in great shape.

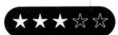

1.2 Indicates a 3-Star or Intermediate Exercise

Inflatable and Foam Roller Symbols

For your convenience, I have included an inflatable and foam roller symbol (see illustration 1.3) that designates – at a quick glance – whether an inflatable or foam roller, or both, is appropriate to use with each exercise. A check mark ✓ indicates the identified roller is appropriate to use and an ✗ indicates it is inappropriate to use. The text below the symbols describes why a particular roller is or is not recommended.

Chapters I - VII

The remainder of this chapter will cover how to begin, when not to exercise, how to monitor your body and adjust workouts depending on how your body feels, etc., and discuss the 10 Tips for A Successful Exercise Program.

Chapter II will introduce you to the inflatable and foam rollers. It will discuss the similarities and differences of the rollers and the most commonly asked questions.

Core Strengthening, Chapter III, includes the latest research regarding why it is so important to strengthen your core muscles. Also learn why traditional sit-ups can cause the abdomen to bulge, weakening the abdominal muscles instead of strengthening them.

The exercises included in Chapter III are considered the 5 Essential Core Strengthening Exercises, because they focus on strengthening the muscles that provide support and stability to your pelvis, hip, spine, and abdomen in a basic, stationary position. In my experience, the majority of the population has weak core muscles, due to pregnancy, weight gain, injury, illness, etc. For this reason, it is imperative to learn how to retrain and strengthen the core muscles in a static position before progressing an exercise program to more advanced or dynamic exercises. Dynamic exercises require a lot of support, strength,

ROLLERS...	
✗	FOAM
✓	INFLATABLE

It is uncomfortable to use a foam roller.

1.3 Inflatable and Foam Roller Symbol - Indicating Roller Type(s) Recommended

> It is imperative to learn how to retrain and strengthen the core muscles in a static position before progressing an exercise program to more advanced or dynamic exercises.

Core Strength Training   **Ch1 Introduction**

After you have become proficient at performing the 5 Essential Core Strengthening Exercises and diaphragmatic breathing you may progress on to higher-level exercises, such as inflatable roller and foam roller exercises.

The mini-workouts are located at the back of your book – you may tear them out, post them on a wall, or take them with you.

1.4 Enclosed 4-color Poster

and stability, such as with running, high impact aerobics, and three to five star foam and inflatable roller exercises.

After you have become proficient at performing the 5 Essential Core Strengthening Exercises and diaphragmatic breathing – this may take 2 to 6 weeks depending on your current physical capability – you may progress on to higher-level exercises (Chapters IV and V).

Any exercise regimen should begin with a good stretching program. The stretching exercises found in Chapter IV will help relieve stress, improve posture, and increase muscle flexibility.

Dynamic Core Strengthening exercises as illustrated in Chapter V will focus on the working relationship of the abdominal, back, diaphragm, pelvic floor and hip muscles. This is by far the largest chapter of the book, so it has been broken down into three parts: upper body exercises, core exercises, and lower body exercises. Even though the chapter separates upper and lower body exercises —all of the exercises will strengthen the core muscles, too.

A flow chart is enclosed at the back of the Strengthening Exercises chapter. You can record your progress on the number of sets and repetitions of each exercise completed, along with your exercise heart rate.

The Mini-Workouts in Chapter VI were designed as a quick reference to the exercises illustrated throughout the book, to give you workout routine ideas, and to provide a variety of workouts for every level of fitness enthusiast – beginner to expert.

The suggested workouts add variety, provide greater strength and endurance gains in less time, and can be used to create more time-intensive and challenging exercise regimens. The mini-workouts are located at the back of your book – you may tear them out, post them on a wall, or take them with you.

Aerobic exercise is an important part of a well-rounded exercise program. Chapter VII will teach you how to calculate your target heart rate and take your pulse, the benefits of aerobic exercise and other forms of physical activity.

The 4-color poster (see illustration 1.4) enclosed at the back of your book includes popular inflatable and foam roller exercises. The Core Strength Training Using Inflatable and Foam Roller Poster can be removed easily from the book, and you can post it in a convenient location for a quick reference to some of the most popular foam and inflatable roller exercises illustrated in this book.

Fourteen stretching, strengthening, and balancing exercises are illustrated on the poster as well as corresponding exercise hints. As in the book, the poster includes the five star exercise rating system and the inflatable and foam roller symbol – indicating the appropriateness of each roller type for each exercise.

10 Tips for a Successful Exercise Program

One of the best pieces of advice I can share with you in regards to exercising properly is to **LISTEN TO YOUR BODY!** If exercise feels good, and you are enjoying what you do, then **LISTEN TO YOUR BODY**, and continue doing what you are doing. If you feel your back arch too much with the Back Extension–Advanced exercise, page 127, or if you are having discomfort or pain with this exercise or any other exercise then you need to **LISTEN TO YOUR BODY** and revise your exercise regimen by reducing intensity, frequency, duration, and/or type of exercise.

"NO PAIN NO GAIN" IS A MYTH. Pain is your body's way of telling you that something is not quite right. Pain will usually lead to swelling, soreness, and more pain. Try a different exercise, reduce your exercise repetitions, frequency, or you may need to stop performing this particular exercise until you can perform it without pain or discomfort.

10 TIPS FOR A SUCCESSFUL EXERCISE PROGRAM

1.
LISTEN TO YOUR BODY

2.
"NO PAIN NO GAIN"
IS A MYTH

3.
QUALITY OF MOVEMENT NOT
QUANTITY OF EXERCISES

4.
FATIGUE CAUSES
MUSCLE SUBSTITUTION

5.
MAINTAIN GOOD POSTURE
WHILE PERFORMING
EACH EXERCISE

6.
ADAPT THE EXERCISE
TO YOUR BODY, NOT YOUR
BODY TO THE EXERCISE

7.
RESUME YOUR EXERCISE
ROUTINE GRADUALLY

8.
CUSTOMIZE YOUR EXERCISE
PROGRAM TO MEET THE
INDIVIDUALIZED NEEDS
OF YOUR OWN BODY

9.
PROGRESS EXERCISES FROM
STATIONARY TO DYNAMIC
AND FROM BASIC
TO ADVANCED

10.
A WELL-ROUNDED EXERCISE
PROGRAM INCLUDES
STRETCHING,
STRENGTHENING, AND
AEROBIC EXERCISES

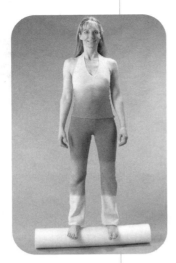

*1.5 Standing Position
on a Foam Roller*

Body size, shape,
body awareness, etc.
can influence your
ability to perform
an exercise.

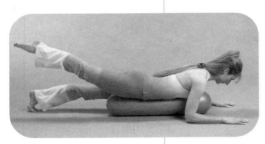

1.6 Booty Buster Leg Raise

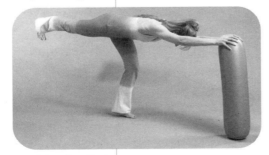

1.7 Standing Plank

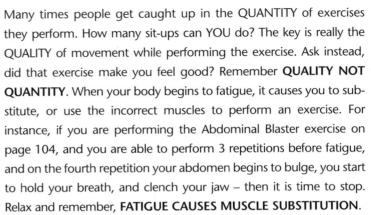

Many times people get caught up in the QUANTITY of exercises they perform. How many sit-ups can YOU do? The key is really the QUALITY of movement while performing the exercise. Ask instead, did that exercise make you feel good? Remember **QUALITY NOT QUANTITY**. When your body begins to fatigue, it causes you to substitute, or use the incorrect muscles to perform an exercise. For instance, if you are performing the Abdominal Blaster exercise on page 104, and you are able to perform 3 repetitions before fatigue, and on the fourth repetition your abdomen begins to bulge, you start to hold your breath, and clench your jaw – then it is time to stop. Relax and remember, **FATIGUE CAUSES MUSCLE SUBSTITUTION**.

MAINTAIN GOOD POSTURE WHILE PERFORMING EACH EXERCISE. Good exercise posture ensures you are working the correct muscles. Exercising with poor posture can cause muscle substitution, meaning you are using the wrong muscle or muscle groups.

Body size, shape, body awareness, etc. can influence your ability to perform an exercise. For example, if you find it difficult to perform the Standing Position on a Foam Roller, illustration 1.5, try one of the kneeling exercises on the inflatable roller, pages 64-78. Or if you are having a difficult time performing push-ups on the inflatable rollers, pages 85 and 56, try the Prone Walkout exercise, page 108, instead. If the Booty Buster Leg Raise exercise, illustration 1.6, becomes easy to do, and you find you are in great shape, try performing the Standing Plank, illustration 1.7. **ADAPT EACH EXERCISE TO YOUR BODY, NOT YOUR BODY TO THE EXERCISE.**

Core Strength Training © *2006 Caroline Corning Creager 1-800-530-6878*

Whether you are fit or not, each individual will require more or less time to strengthen their core muscles appropriately. **RESUME YOUR EXERCISE ROUTINE GRADUALLY and CUSTOMIZE YOUR EXERCISE PROGRAM TO MEET THE INDIVIDUALIZED NEEDS OF YOUR OWN BODY.**

Research has shown that it is best to begin strengthening your core muscles in a stationary position. Dynamic exercises are more advanced and can overload your muscular and balance systems if initiated too soon. **PROGRESS EXERCISES FROM STATIONARY TO DYNAMIC AND FROM BASIC TO MORE ADVANCED.**

1. Begin with the 5 Essential Core Exercises on pages 24-28. Once you are able to hold the Transverse Abdominis exercise for 15 – 20 seconds, ten times in a row, proceed to #2.

2. Progress to stretching exercises and exercises rated with one through three stars (* – ***) on the inflatable and foam roller. Maintain a neutral spine with all exercises: a position where the back is not arched or flat, it is somewhere in between.

3. Proceed to basic dynamic core strengthening exercises on the inflatable or foam roller (* – ***).

4. Add advanced dynamic core strengthening exercises on the inflatable or foam rollers (**** – *****), (see illustration 1.8) when you are able to follow all of the 10 Tips To A Successful Exercise Program.

> Research has shown that it is best to begin strengthening your core muscles in a stationary position.

A WELL-ROUNDED EXERCISE PROGRAM INCLUDES STRETCHING, STRENGTHENING, AND AEROBIC EXERCISES. Please read chapters IV, V, and VII respectively for more information on these different types of exercise. Begin with the exercises depicted in the Core Strengthening chapter as recommended on pages 22–29, and then progress to aerobic, and inflatable and foam roller stretching and strengthening exercises. Follow the 10 TIPS TO A SUCCESSFUL EXERCISE PROGRAM, and enjoy your exercise journey.

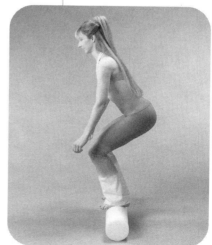

1.8 Standing Squat on Foam Roller

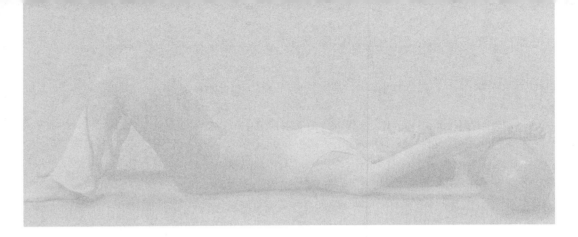

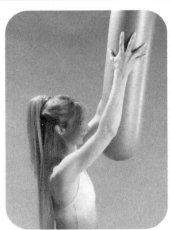

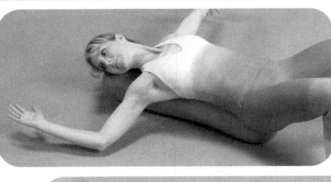

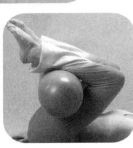

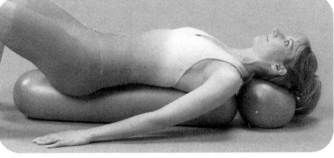

What are inflatable and foam rollers?

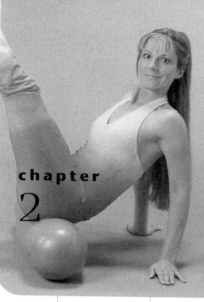

Inflatable Rollers

An inflatable roller is a cross between a fitness ball and a foam roller. It is cylindrical in shape like a foam roller and is made from burst-resistant vinyl, holding up to 440 pounds, like a fitness ball. You could say an inflatable roller is a ball squeezed down into a tube shape.

The versatility of the inflatable roller make it a great addition to any home gym, health club, fitness class, or therapy clinic. The inflatable roller is a great exercise tool because you can work on balance, body awareness, flexibility, and strengthen the abs, obliques, and core muscle groups all at the same time.

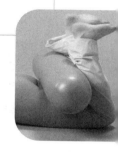

> An inflatable roller is a cross between a fitness ball and a foam roller.

Tracey Olson, BS, and ACSM group fitness instructor, remembers, "I was able to transition my ball strengthening class easily to the inflatable roller. Our club members not only told me how much they enjoyed the inflatable rollers, but that they couldn't believe how much their core muscles were being targeted with this new piece of equipment."

The inflatable roller is so versatile you can inflate it with a small air pump, deflate it easily, and pack it in a suitcase or gym bag. Brett Pruitt, MS, Exercise Physiologist, and ACE Certified Personal Trainer and Exam Prep Instructor, says

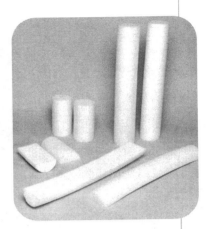
2.1 Foam Rollers

that the inflatable roller "is fun, inviting, light, and portable. It is a great tool for personal trainers and their clients – who work at the gym, home, or office setting – and want to further enhance their stability or functional core strengthening program."

Foam Rollers

Foam rollers are cylindrical in shape, lightweight, durable – holding more than 300 pounds of weight – and vary in length, circumference, and density. Most foam rollers are comprised of polyethylene. Polyethylene is also found in running shoes and medical appliances.

> Foam rollers are cylindrical in shape, lightweight, durable – holding more than 300 pounds of weight – and vary in length, circumference, and density.

The foam roller's design provides sensory motor challenges in two planes and enhances balance reactions, body awareness, muscle reeducation, motor planning, dynamic strengthening, and neural and muscular flexibility.

Although foam roller lengths, and circumferences can vary (see illustration 2.1), for the sake of simplicity, the majority of references to the foam roller in this book are to a 3 foot long (90 centimeter) 6 inch (15 centimeter) diameter roller. In several instances, pages 50, 64–67, 69–78, 144 and 146, I mention that a half-roller, 3 feet long (90 centimeter) 3 inch diameter (7.5 centimeters), is optimal for the exercises.

Frequently Asked Questions About Inflatable and Foam Rollers

How do I inflate an inflatable roller?
- An air compressor or hand pump can be used to inflate the inflatable roller
- Withdraw the plug from roller (see illustration 2.2)
- Insert the pump nozzle into the opening of the roller
- Inflate the roller to its maximum diameter, 7 inches (17.5 centimeters) or less
- Place the plug back in roller

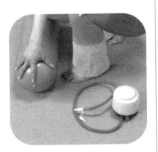
2.2 To Inflate Roller–
Withdraw Plug From Roller
And Insert Pump Nozzle

Ch2 Rollers   **Core Strength Training** *© 2006 Caroline Corning Creager 1-800-530-6878*

Will an inflatable roller burst if it is punctured?

No, the inflatable rollers are burst resistant. This means if you puncture it with a sharp object it will deflate slowly and not burst.

> Inflatable rollers are burst resistant.

What is the best way to clean inflatable and foam rollers?

For home use, clean the inflatable rollers with soap and water and in the clinic, clean them with the same disinfectant you would use on the plinth. For the foam roller, I highly recommend you place a vinyl sleeve over it. Since the foam rollers are porous, the sleeve is easier to keep clean. Cloth sleeves are inexpensive and you can purchase one by calling Orthopedic Physical Therapy Products at 800-367-7393.

How long will inflatable and foam rollers last?

Although inflatable rollers were only recently introduced to the market, they are made from the same material as the Swiss Balls, or large fitness balls. I have had clients and clinics report that their fitness ball has lasted more than 10 years.

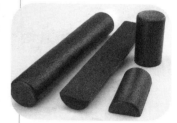

2.3 Axis®Foam Rollers are molded foam and last longer than the traditional porous foam rollers.

I have several foam rollers that are at least 8 years old. Some foam rollers are more porous than others. The less porous foam rollers, such as the Axis® Roller, tend to last longer and maintain their shape better.

Are the inflatable and foam rollers safe for people with latex allergies?

Yes, the inflatable roller is a safe product for individuals who are sensitive or allergic to latex. The inflatable rollers are made from vinyl, not latex, and foam rollers are traditionally made from polyethelene.

> The inflatable roller is a safe product for individuals who are sensitive or allergic to latex.

Are all the inflatable rollers the same size and shape?

The Core Challenge Roller® and the FitBall® Roller are Italian-made rollers that measure 30 inches (75 centimeters) in length and 7 inches (17.5 centimeters) in diameter.

The AirRoller® is an Australian-made inflatable roller and it is 29.5 inches (90 centimeters) long and 27.5 inches (70 centimeters) in diameter.

2.4 Cervical Stabilization

The inflatable roller is not as long as the foam roller. How will my tall clients fit on the roller?

Although the inflatable roller is shorter than the traditional foam roller, a soft inflatable foam ball can be placed under the head (see illustration 2.4) or the pelvis (see illustration 2.5). The ball supports the head or pelvis while the roller supports the body, accommodating a taller person.

Why shouldn't I stand on an inflatable roller?

2.5 Pelvic Stabilization

Standing on an inflatable roller is not recommended for anyone – therapy clinic patients and fitness club members alike. Due to its pliable and dynamic nature, the inflatable roller is dangerous to stand on.

Is it safe to stand on a foam roller?

Yes, it is safe to stand on a foam roller if you follow proper precautions. You should never wear shoes when standing on the round surface of the foam roller. Your body awareness is decreased and your foot is unable to conform to the roller when you wear shoes.

You should always have a designated spotter when you perform any standing exercises on a foam roller, in an area free of clutter. If standing on a round foam roller is too difficult, try standing on a half-round roller with the flat surface up.

While it is possible to use a swimming noodle for specific exercises, optimal core strength training on land requires a foam roller approximately 6 inches, 15 centimeters, in diameter.

Can I use a 'swimming noodle' instead of a foam roller?

While it is possible to use a swimming noodle for specific exercises, optimal core strength training on land requires a foam roller approximately 6 inches, 15 centimeters, in diameter. The larger diameter of a foam roller allows less of your body to make contact with the floor and therefore challenges the body more.

      Core Strength Training © 2006 Caroline Corning Creager 1-800-530-6878

Is the inflatable roller better to use than the foam roller or vice versa?

Both inflatable rollers and foam rollers are excellent tools to promote core strength, body awareness, and balance. Each type of roller has properties unique to it, therefore, I do not believe one style of roller is superior to the other.

Roller Exercise Tips

• Perform exercises away from furniture and sharp objects.

• Never hold your breath when performing an exercise. Always exhale when the exercise is most difficult. For example, exhale as you raise your knees to your chest. Inhale as you lower your knees (see illustrations 2.6 and 2.7).

• The following may damage an inflatable roller: sharp objects (belt buckles, jewelry, staples, cat claws etc.), heat sources (direct sunlight, heaters, fireplaces, etc.), and inflating the inflatable roller beyond the maximum diameter.

• If at any time an exercise causes discomfort or pain, revise your exercise regimen by reducing intensity, frequency, duration, and/or type of exercise. If any of these symptoms persist, discontinue the exercise.

• The closer the rollers are to the body, the easier it is to maintain a neutral spine. Make exercises more difficult by rolling the rollers further away from the body and decreasing points of stable contact.

• If it is too uncomfortable to lay on a foam roller, place a towel on the roller between your back and the roller.

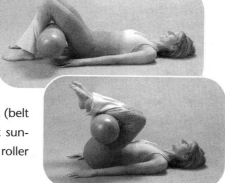

2.6 Lower Abdominal Crunch - Exhale

2.7 Lower Abdominal Crunch - Inhale

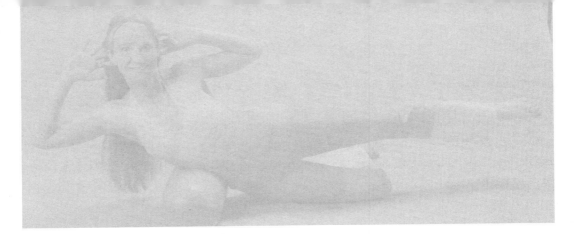

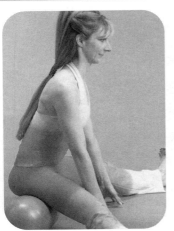

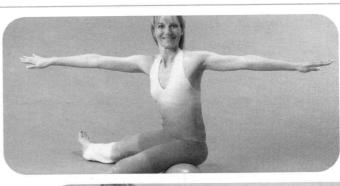

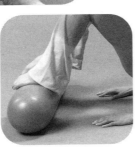

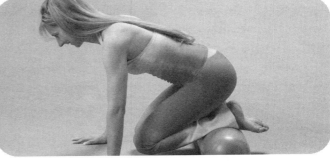

Core Strength Training *© 2006 Caroline Corning Creager 1-800-530-6878*

Core Strengthening

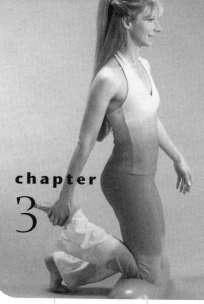

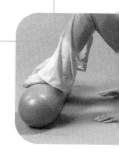

Does your lower abdomen bulge? Does your lower back or hip hurt? Do you leak urine when you cough, sneeze, or jump? Are you prone to injuries with exercise, lifting, or physical exertion? If you have answered yes to one or more of these questions, your core muscles are most likely weak.

The exercises illustrated in this chapter will focus on the working relationship of the abdominal, back, diaphragm, pelvic floor, and hip muscles. It is very important to learn how to use and properly strengthen these "core" muscles before progressing with an exercise program. To better understand the important role the abdominal, back, diaphragm, hip, and pelvic floor muscles play in providing support and stability to your pelvis, spine, and abdomen, it is important to begin by identifying where all of these muscles are located.

Think of a 3-dimensional cylinder—at the top of the cylinder is the diaphragm muscle, the front side is the abdominal muscles, the bottom side is the pelvic floor muscles, and the back side of the cylinder is the back and hip muscles (Richardson, Jull, Hodges, and Hides, 1998.), see illustration 3.1 on the next page.

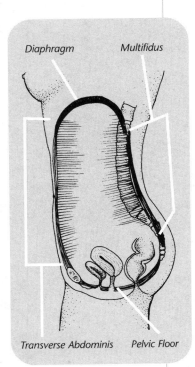

Diaphragm

Multifidus

Transverse Abdominis

Pelvic Floor

3.1 Core Stability Muscles

Diaphragm

The dome-shaped diaphragm muscle is the largest and primary breathing muscle. It separates the lungs from the abdominal cavity. When you breathe in, or inhale, the diaphragm muscle contracts and moves down, compressing the abdominal contents and increasing (intra-abdominal) pressure on your bladder, bowel, and pelvic floor muscles. If the muscles are weak, and cannot contract <u>up against pressure</u>, urine leaks out. This is why women or men with weak pelvic floor muscles may leak urine when coughing, sneezing, jumping etc.

During exhalation, or breathing out, the diaphragm muscle returns to its dome shape causing a decrease in intra-abdominal pressure. It is easiest to contract pelvic floor muscles when there is less resistance or pressure. Pelvic floor muscles therefore must first be strengthened *after* or *during exhalation*, when the intra-abdominal pressure has decreased. When pelvic floor muscles become stronger, they can then be strengthened against intra-abdominal pressure, as with inhalation.

Diaphragmatic breathing, also known as belly breathing, is the correct form of breathing. Chest and shoulder breathing are very common methods of breathing despite the fact they are incorrect. Imagine the tension that can develop in the chest or shoulder region when you are breathing incorrectly, since the average person breathes in and out 23,040 times per day!

Diaphragmatic breathing helps reduce muscular tension, promotes relaxation, and restores the working relationship between the pelvic floor, back, and abdominal muscles. In order to effectively engage the transverse abdominis, multifidus, or pelvic floor muscles, you must be able to disassociate the diaphragm muscle from them. Hence the importance of learning how to breath diaphragmatically as illustrated on page 29.

Core Strength Training *© 2006 Caroline Corning Creager 1-800-530-6878*

Transverse Abdominis and Multifidus Muscles

The *transverse abdominis and multifidus muscles,* part of the abdominal and back family muscles respectively, have been identified as being key muscles in stabilizing the spine (Richardson, Jull, Hodges, Hides, 1998). The transverse abdominis and multifidus muscles are the abdominal and back muscles identified on the previous illustration.

When the transverse abdominis muscle contracts, the abdomen moves toward the spine. This muscle acts as a corset to the abdominal contents, and assists with the stabilization of the spine. The contraction of the multifidus muscle is less discernable, however it may be felt on both sides of the spine in the lower back region. This muscle keeps the spine in proper alignment, prevents excessive movement in the spine, and of course works with the transverse abdominis muscle in stabilizing the spine.

The transverse abdominis muscle has been shown to assist in the contraction of the multifidus muscle and vice versa (Richardson and Jull, 1995). In other words, if you are having a difficult time determining where the multifidus muscles are or how to contract them, try tightening your transverse abdominis muscle as on page 26, and it will automatically contract the multifidus muscle.

Furthermore, Richardson et. al., 2002, found that the contraction of the transverse abdominis muscle significantly reduces the laxity, or increases the stiffness, of the sacroiliac joint. This means the sacroiliac joint, a common area of pain and instability, is stabilized with the contraction of the transverse abdominis muscle.

Research has shown that with minimal instruction people can alter the muscle activity of the abdominal muscles when performing a sit-up (Karst, G. and Willett, G., 2004). Sit-ups, unless otherwise

The *transverse abdominis and multifidus muscles,* part of the abdominal and back family muscles respectively, have been identified as being key muscles in stabilizing the spine (Richardson, Jull, Hodges, Hides, 1998).

The sacroiliac joint, a common area of pain and instability, is stabilized with the contraction of the transverse abdominis muscle.

Research has shown that with minimal instruction people can alter the muscle activity of the abdominal muscles when performing a sit-up (Karst, G. and Willett, G., 2004).

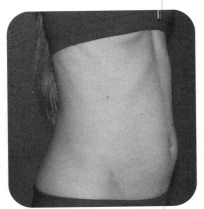

3.2 Relaxed Transverse Abdominis Muscle

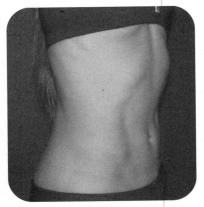

3.3 Contracted Transverse Abdominis Muscle

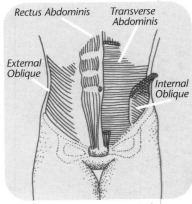

3.4 Four layers of Abdominal muscles

instructed, strengthen the most superficial layer of abdominal muscles. If you perform a sit-up when your deepest abdominal muscle layer, the transverse abdominis muscle, is weak, it is unable to act as a corset and function as a stabilizer to the abdomen.

Consequently, when performing a sit-up, the transverse abdominis muscle – when weak – will cause the abdomen to bulge out and prevent the rectus abdominis muscle from tightening in an optimal position. When the transverse abdominis muscles becomes stronger, or is engaged while doing a sit-up, it is able to function as a corset and prevent the abdomen from bulging. Illustration 3.2 depicts the abdomen when the transverse abdominis muscle is relaxed, and illustration 3.3 depicts the transverse abdominis muscle when it is contracted.

Notice how the back is less arched after the transverse abdominis muscle is tightened, illustration 3.3. Core trunk posture correction, described below, has been shown to occur as well with pelvic floor reeducation and pelvic floor muscle strengthening exercises (Bemelmans, 1997).

The secret to a successful abdominal strengthening program, and ridding yourself of an "abdominal pooch", is to strengthen the muscles from the inner to the outermost layers. The four different abdominal muscles, from inner to outermost layers, are the transverse abdominis, internal oblique, external oblique, and rectus abdominis muscles, illustration 3.4.

Photographs were taken of each of these muscles in a standing position. Each specialized muscle function and corresponding photograph are summarized and depicted below.

Transverse abdominis – Innermost layer. Works in synergy (together) with the back (multifidus muscle) and pelvic floor muscles. Assists with stabilizing, or controlling movement of the abdomen/spine before trunk, arms or legs are moved. The waist narrows and the lower abdomen draws inward when the transverse abdominis muscle contracts, similar to the action of a corset. To feel the transverse abdominis muscle, place your fingers just inside your hipbones.

Contract the transverse abdominis as instructed on page 26. You should feel the muscle tighten beneath your fingers. In the event you are unable to feel the transverse abdominis muscle contract beneath your fingers, try performing a Kegel as illustrated on page 27. If your abdomen bulges or you feel yourself bearing down, try again, you are contracting the muscle incorrectly.

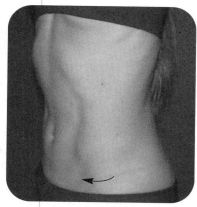

*3.5 Transverse Abdominis –
Innermost Layer*

Internal and External Obliques – Middle layers. These muscles work together to assist with rotation, side bending and breathing, such as with the *Sideways Crunch*, page 98, *Tummy Trimmin Trunk Curl - Beginner*, page 100, and *Diaphragmatic Breathing*, page 29. The external oblique muscle assists with bowel movements by pulling the ribcage down and in. The internal oblique is difficult to feel because it is located beneath the external oblique. To feel the external oblique muscle, place your hands on your hips. Contract the transverse abdominis muscle as instructed on page 26, gently draw your lower abdomen in further. You should feel your waist widen, pushing out into your hands.

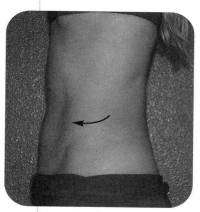

*3.6 Internal and External
Obliques–Middle Layers*

Rectus abdominis – Outer most layer. Flexes the trunk, as with a sit-up. This muscle may separate down the middle during intense weight lifting or pregnancy and cause a diastasis recti, a separation of the connective tissue attaching to the rectus abdominis muscle. To feel your rectus abdominis muscle, lie on your back with knees bent. Place your hands in the middle of your abdomen. Lift your head off the floor. You should feel your abdomen tighten underneath your fingers.

All of these muscles become stretched or weakened during pregnancy, after gaining weight or long periods of inactivity. Therefore it becomes paramount to learn how to contract each of these muscles,

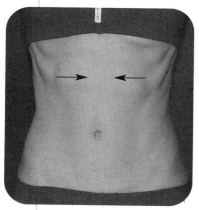

*3.7 Rectus Abdominis –
Outermost Layer*

Once you are able to strengthen your abdominal muscles correctly, you will be on your way to developing a sleek, strong, and stabile abdomen.

learn their specialized muscle function, and strengthen them appropriately. Once you are able to strengthen your abdominal muscles correctly, you will be on your way to developing a sleek, strong, and stabile abdomen.

Pelvic Floor

The *pelvic floor muscles* make up the base of the cylinder, as illustrated in 3.1 and 3.8 and contribute to trunk stability. The pelvic floor muscles are the only muscles in our body that work in a transverse plane and function as a load bearing muscle group – supporting the pelvic organs.

The pelvic floor muscles are the only muscles in our body that work in a transverse plane and function as a load bearing muscle group – supporting the pelvic organs.

Interestingly enough, researchers have found a working relationship between the pelvic floor and the abdominal muscles. The pelvic floor muscles have been shown to work in unison with all the abdominal muscles, – internal oblique, external oblique, rectus abdominis, and most importantly the transverse abdominis muscle. (Sapsford, et. al; 2001).

Kegel exercises, developed by Dr. Arnold Kegel in the 1940s, are often recommended to strengthen the pelvic floor muscles. Strong pelvic floor muscles are imperative for support of pelvic organs, sexual sensation, and sphincteric control for continence of bowel and bladder. The Agency for Health Care Policy and Research, 1994, reports that 87% of people who perform pelvic floor exercises significantly reduce or eliminate incontinence.

Men and women must strengthen the pelvic floor in order to achieve or maintain core strength. As mentioned previously, the pelvic floor muscles must be able to work with or against the intra-abdominal pressure changes caused by the diaphragm muscle.

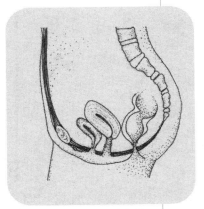

3.8 Pelvic Floor

Hip

The abdominal, pelvic floor, and hips all have a common factor – they have muscles that attach to the hip/pelvic bones (also known as the innominate bone). Hence, abdominal and pelvic floor weakness can affect the hips and vice versa.

Leetun et. al., 2004, reported that "athletes who experienced an injury over the course of the season generally demonstrated lower core stability measures (hip weakness) than those who did not."

Furthermore they found that athletes who had strong hip external rotators and abductors – hip muscles that stabilize the hip – did not sustain injuries to the knees or ankles.

The abdominal, pelvic floor, and hips all have a common factor – they have muscles that attach to the hip/pelvic bones (also known as the innominate bone).

Lower Core and Upper Core

When I think of the core muscles, I think of the body as having a lower core (abdomen, lower back, pelvic floor, and hip) and an upper core (upper back, scapulae, and neck). If you strengthen the transverse abdominis muscle it will certainly improve your posture, as noted in photographs 3.2 versus 3.3. However, to further improve the upper core, you will need to strengthen the scapular muscles, see illustration 3.9, and the deep cervical (neck) muscles, see illustration 3.10. For this reason, The 5 Essential Core Exercises include exercises for the scapular and cervical muscles.

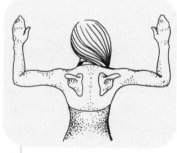

3.9 Scapular Stabilizer

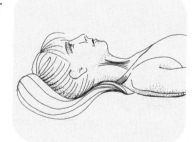

3.10 Neck Stabilizer

5 Essential Core Exercises

As basic exercises –
The 5 Essential Core Exercises –
are mastered you may
progress on to more
dynamic exercises on the
inflatable or foam roller.

As you can see, the diaphragm, transverse abdominis, multifidus, pelvic floor and hip muscles all work together very closely. *Core Strength Training Using Inflatable and Foam Rollers* focuses on strengthening your core muscles first. As basic exercises – *The 5 Essential Core Exercises* – are mastered you may progress on to more dynamic exercises on the inflatable or foam roller.

The 5 Essential Core Exercises include: *Neck Stabilizer, Scapular Stabilizer, Transverse Abdominis Raise, Kegel,* and the *Hip Stabilizer.* A *Diaphragmatic Breathing* exercise is also included, because you will need to learn how to use the diaphragm muscle independently of the abdominal, back, and pelvic floor muscles.

If you have weakness in your mid–
back or scapular region it will affect the
position of your neck and your 'core' – causing
muscular imbalances that may lead to
weakness in your abdomen, back,
or pelvic floor.

If you have weakness in your mid–back or scapular region (between the shoulder blades), it will affect the position of your neck and your 'core' – causing muscular imbalances that may lead to weakness in your abdomen, back, or pelvic floor. For this reason, I decided it was important to include basic exercises for the deep neck and scapular muscles.

Gradually increase the HOLD time and/or repetitions of each exercise, if it is appropriate for the exercise, as your strength and endurance improve. Keep in mind it is not important how many repetitions of each exercise you perform; it is important to perform the exercise properly without substitution of inappropriate muscles. Remember the phrases, **Quality Not Quantity** and **Fatigue Causes Muscle Substitution**, when performing the *5 Essential Core Exercises*. The *5 Essential Core Exercises* can be found on pages 24-28 and 168.

Keep in mind it is not important
how many repetitions of each
exercise you perform; it is
important to perform the exercise
properly without substitution
of inappropriate muscles.

5 Essential Core Exercises + Diaphragmatic Breathing   page

core exercises + breathing

Exercises

© 2006 Caroline Corning Creager 1-800-530-6878 **Core Strength Training**   **Ch3 Core Strengthening**

★☆☆☆☆

Neck Stabilizer

TARGET AREAS:
Deep muscles of neck.

hold:
5–20 seconds

repeat:
2–10 times

frequency:
2–3 times per day, everyday

HELPFUL HINTS:

- This is a very gentle exercise. If you move your neck with this exercise you will recruit the stronger superficial muscles of the neck.

- This exercise may be performed lying down and later in a sitting position.

BENEFITS:

This exercise improves neck posture, and helps stabilize the cervical (neck) spine. It strengthens the deep cervical muscles – the longus capitus and longus coli.

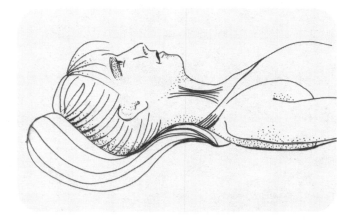

INSTRUCTION:

Lie on back with knees bent. Relax shoulders and neck. Take a relaxed breath in and out. Now without breathing in, slowly and gently activate the deep neck muscles by **imagining** you are flattening out the curve in your neck. Hold, breathe lightly. Relax the deep neck muscles slowly.

Scapular Stabilizer

★☆☆☆☆

TARGET AREA: *Mid back.*

hold:
5–20 seconds

repeat:
2–10 times

frequency:
2–3 times per day, everyday, or every time phone rings

BENEFITS:

This exercise improves posture and helps stabilize the shoulder blades. It also strengthens the middle and lower trapezius muscles.

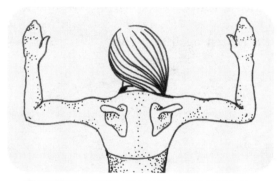

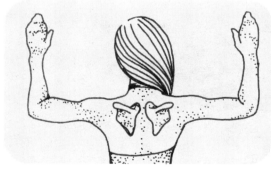

INSTRUCTION:

Lie on abdomen with head placed on a small towel roll. Place hands on floor at a 90-degree angle (or less) from body. Relax shoulders and neck. Take a relaxed breath in and out. Now without breathing in, slowly and gently draw the lower abdomen in towards the spine and the shoulder blades down and in – as if squeezing the shoulder blades together. Hold, breathe lightly. Relax the abdomen and shoulder blades gradually. Progress exercise by performing it in sitting or standing positions.

HELPFUL HINTS:

- This is a very gentle exercise. If you pull your shoulders up toward your ears, the incorrect (upper trapezius) muscle will be recruited.

- This exercise may be progressed by raising the arms off the floor. Keep shoulder blades down and in as you raise the arms off the floor.

Ch3 Core Strengthening

Transverse Abdominis Raise

TARGET AREAS:
Deep abdominal muscles.

hold:
5–20 seconds

repeat:
2–10 times

frequency:
2–3 times per day, everyday, or every time phone rings

HELPFUL HINTS:

■ This is a very gentle exercise.

■ This exercise may be performed lying down, standing and later in sitting position.

■ Avoid movement of the trunk or pelvis, and avoid using inner thigh, and buttock muscles when performing exercise.

BENEFITS:

This exercise improves posture, abdominal, and pelvic floor strength, and helps stabilize the spine. It also promotes the working relationship between the abdominal, back, and pelvic floor muscles. This exercise strengthens the transverse abdominis muscle against gravity.

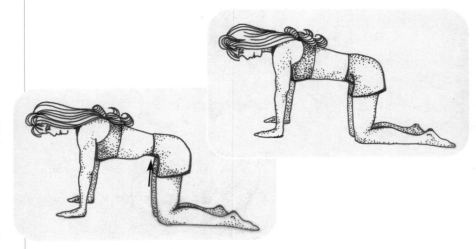

INSTRUCTION:

Kneel. Lean forward and place hands on floor. Align shoulders and hands, and hips and knees. Maintain head alignment with body, and a neutral spine position. Take a relaxed breath in and out. Now without breathing in, slowly and gently draw the lower abdomen in towards the spine. Hold, breathe lightly. Relax the abdomen gradually. If you find this exercise difficult to perform, do it while lying on your side or on your abdomen. Neutral spine: A position where the back is not arched or flat, it is somewhere in between.

Core Strength Training © 2006 Caroline Corning Creager 1-800-530-6878

Kegel

★★☆☆☆

BENEFITS:

The Kegel improves pelvic floor support and muscle strength and endurance, as with maintaining good posture, standing/sitting throughout the day. It will also help you gain awareness of how to use and coordinate the pelvic floor muscles.

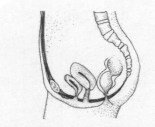

Pelvic Floor at rest

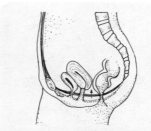

Pelvic Floor pulled up and In

INSTRUCTION:

Lie down on back with knees bent and feet shoulder-width apart. Take a relaxed breath in and out. Now without breathing in, slowly draw the pelvic floor muscles up and in as if you are attempting to stop urine flow. Inhale. Hold this position for 3 seconds. Gradually relax the pelvic floor muscles for 6 seconds.

Exercise Progression: Once you have mastered this exercise, progress to doing the exercise sitting, standing, or squatting. Avoid movement or contraction of the upper abdominal, buttock, and/or inner thigh muscles while performing exercise. If you have difficulty contracting pelvic floor muscles, try this exercise lying on your side.

TARGET AREAS:
Pelvic floor and sphincter muscles.

hold:
3 seconds, gradually increase to 20 seconds

repeat:
3–10 times

frequency:
3 times daily

HELPFUL HINTS:

- Your relaxation period should be twice as long as your hold time, until you approach a 10 second hold.

- Avoid movement or contraction of the upper abdominal, buttock, and/or inner thigh muscles while performing exercise.

Ch3 Core Strengthening

5

★☆☆☆☆

Hip Stabilizer

TARGET AREAS:

Hip muscles.

hold:
2 seconds

repeat:
3–10

frequency:
2–3 times a day

HELPFUL HINTS:

- Avoid rolling hips forward or backward.
- Keep a straight line between ears, shoulders, hips, and ankles.

BENEFITS:

This exercise will help strengthen and stabilize the hip— most specifically the gluteus medius (side of hip) muscle. The gluteus medius muscle keeps the pelvis level with walking or running.

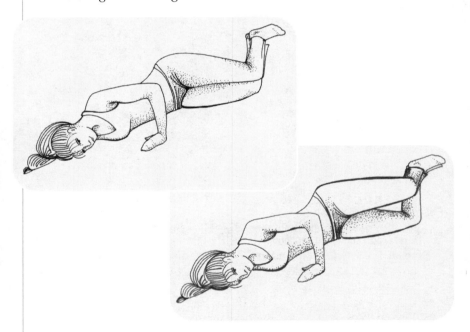

INSTRUCTION:

Lie on side with knees bent at a 90-degree angle. Take a relaxed breath in and out. Now without breathing in, slowly and gently draw the lower abdomen in towards the spine. Keeping heels together raise knees as far as possible without any hip movement. Lower knees. Repeat on opposite side.

Ch3 Core Strengthening

Diaphragmatic Breathing

★☆☆☆☆

TARGET AREA:

Diaphragm.

BENEFITS:

To reduce muscular tension and use of incorrect breathing muscles. To promote relaxation and improve breathing pattern.

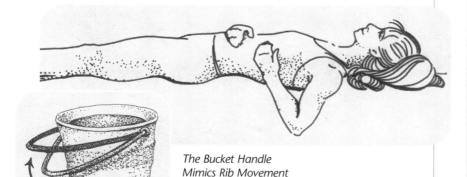

The Bucket Handle Mimics Rib Movement

hold:
inhale for 3 seconds, exhale for 3 seconds

repeat:
30–60 seconds

frequency:
5 times per day, or whenever you feel tense

To determine which type of breathing pattern you use, gently rest one hand on your abdomen and one on your chest. Where do you feel movement? If you feel your abdomen rising into your hand, you are most likely a diaphragmatic breather. If you do not feel any movement in your abdomen and lower ribs, you will need to re-train your breathing muscles.

INSTRUCTION:

Loosen clothing, belts, or remove any other item that restricts the abdomen or causes irritation. Lie on back in a quiet environment and assume a comfortable position – the back is not arched or flat, it is somewhere in between. Relax jaw, place tongue on roof of mouth, and slightly separate teeth. Inhale through nose for 3 seconds allowing lower rib cage to flare up and out like a bucket handle when raised (see illustration). Exhale through nose or mouth for 3 seconds, as abdomen relaxes and ribs lower.

HELPFUL HINTS:

- Avoid elevating chest or shoulders while inhaling.

- The time breathing in should equal the time spent breathing out.

- Neutral spine: A position where the back is not arched or flat, it is somewhere in between.

29

Ch3 Core Strengthening

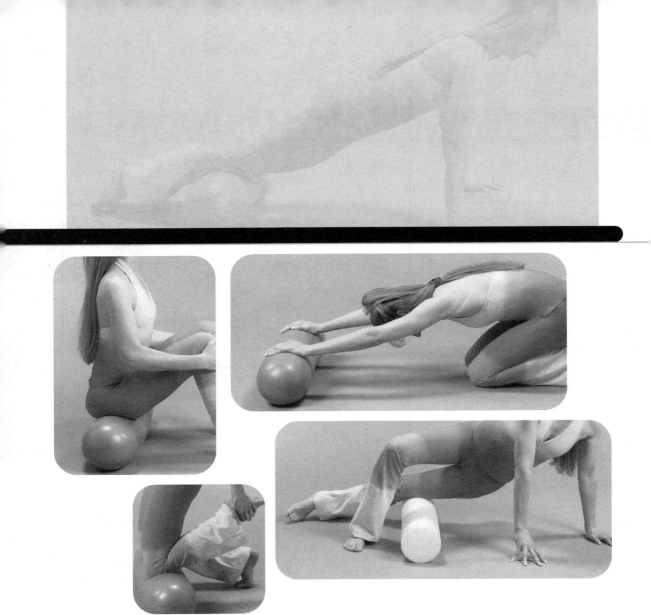

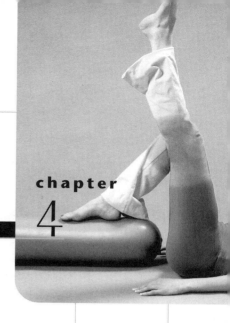

Stretching
Techniques

In our present day society, it is difficult not to become caught up in a fast paced, busy lifestyle that predisposes us to stress and muscle tension.

Tension builds up in our muscles while driving, talking on the phone, or sitting at a computer terminal. These activities cause individual muscle fibers to shorten, decreasing flexibility, and increasing the likelihood of injury.

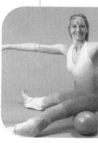

Stretching exercises relieve stress, improve posture, and increase flexibility in tight muscles. Stretching techniques are not complicated, yet there is definitely a proper and improper way to stretch.

To properly stretch a muscle, maintain a slow, static (motionless) stretch. Bouncing or sudden stretching of a muscle triggers a reflex contraction in the muscle being stretched. This contraction is referred to as the myotactic reflex or stretch reflex. The stretch reflex protects our muscles from being overstretched or injured. Bouncing while stretching is therefore counterproductive and may lead to your muscle being overstretched or injured. Watch your cat or dog, they stretch in a slow, sustained motion without any bouncing!

Ch4 Stretching

Proper stretching techniques are essential to effectively increase the length of the muscle and surrounding tissue. Stretching exercises should be performed 15 – 20 minutes before exercising and once again thereafter (Smith, 1994). Stretches may be performed daily, or every other day.

The following guidelines are adapted from: The Warm Up Procedure: To Stretch or Not to Stretch. A Brief Review, by Craig Smith (1994).

1. Avoid bouncing.
2. Slowly stretch into level of tolerance, not pain.
3. Do not hold your breath. Exhale while stretching.
4. Hold stretch for 15 – 20 seconds.
5. Release stretch slowly.
6. Repeat stretch 3 – 5 times.
7. Repeat stretch on both sides of the body.

Stretching Exercises

Stretching

Exercises

1

★☆☆☆☆

Chest Stretch

TARGET AREAS:

Chest and shoulder muscles.

hold:
20 seconds

repeat:
3 times

frequency:
daily

HELPFUL HINTS:

- Head should be supported on roller.
- Vary your arm position for optimal chest and shoulder muscle lengthening.

BENEFITS:

Rounded-shoulder posture is very common. This stretch will elongate or lengthen the chest and shoulder muscles improving posture.

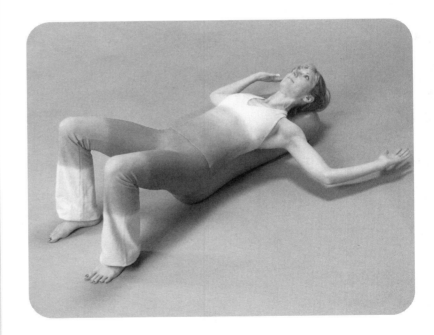

INSTRUCTION:

Lie on side with knees bent. Roll back onto roller with feet flat on floor. Raise arms to 90 degrees and bend elbows to 90 degrees with palms facing up. Hold. Alternate arm position each day you stretch; one day stretch at 45 and 90 degree angles and the next, place the arms at 60 and 120 degree angles.

Core Strength Training © 2006 Caroline Corning Creager 1-800-530-6878

Axillary Stretch

★☆☆☆☆

BENEFITS:

Rounded-shoulder posture is very common. This stretch will elongate or lengthen the chest and shoulder muscles improving posture.

TARGET AREAS:

Axillary nerves and shoulder and chest muscles.

hold:
20 seconds

repeat:
3 times

frequency:
daily

HELPFUL HINTS:

■ Head should be supported on roller.

■ Vary your arm position for optimal chest and shoulder muscle lengthening.

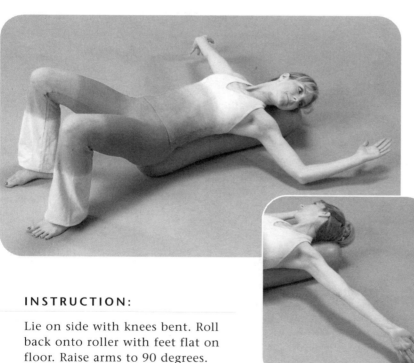

INSTRUCTION:

Lie on side with knees bent. Roll back onto roller with feet flat on floor. Raise arms to 90 degrees. Bend left elbow to 90 degrees and straighten right arm; both with palms facing up. Bent right wrist back so fingers point toward floor. Rotate head to right. Return to starting position and repeat with opposite side.

Ch4 Stretching

★☆☆☆☆

Shoulder Stretch

TARGET AREAS:
Shoulder muscles.

hold:
20 seconds

repeat:
3 times

frequency:
daily

HELPFUL HINTS:

- Avoid rounding back.
- If kneeling or bending knees causes knee discomfort, place roller on table and follow directions as above.

BENEFITS:

To elongate the muscles located in shoulders and upper trunk.

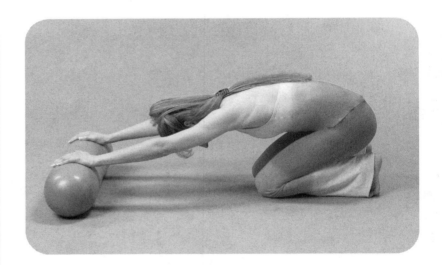

INSTRUCTION:

Kneel. Place roller in front of body and hands on top of roller. Lean forward and roll roller away from body. Lower head so ears are between straight arms.

Back Massage

★☆☆☆☆

BENEFITS:

To improve range of motion in joints and circulation in back muscles.

INSTRUCTION: step one

Lie on side. Place roller horizontal to body next to upper back. Roll back onto roller with knees bent. Place feet flat on the floor. Inhale. Place unclasped hands behind head.

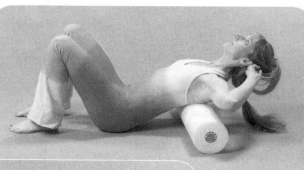

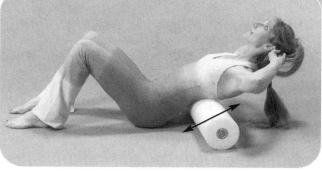

INSTRUCTION: step two

Exhale. Gently draw lower abdomen in toward spine. Roll body up and down roller. Keep body relaxed.

ROLLERS...

✓ FOAM

The firmness provides a better stretch.

✓ INFLATABLE

It is more comfortable to lie on an inflatable foam roller.

TARGET AREAS:
Neck and back.

hold:
20 seconds

repeat:
3 times

frequency:
daily

HELPFUL HINTS:

■ Avoid arching back or pulling on neck with hands.

■ Ribs should remain stationary throughout exercise. If ribs "pop" up, you have lowered head and elbows too far.

Ch4 Stretching

exercise

5

★☆☆☆☆

Mid-Back Stretch

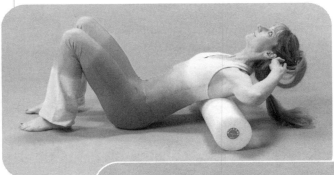

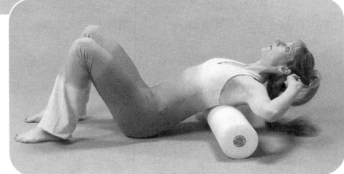

ROLLERS...

✓ FOAM

✓ INFLATABLE

The firmness of a foam roller provides a better stretch.

TARGET AREAS:

Mid-back joints.

hold:
20 seconds

repeat:
3 times

frequency:
daily

HELPFUL HINTS:

- Avoid arching back or pulling on neck with hands.
- Ribs should remain stationary throughout exercise. If ribs "pop" up, you have lowered head and elbows too far.

BENEFITS:

To improve range of motion in mid-back. The mid-back can become very stiff since the ribs stabilize this region and prevent motion.

INSTRUCTION:

Lie on side. Place roller horizontal to body next to upper back. Roll back onto roller with knees bent. Place feet flat on the floor. Inhale. Place unclasped hands behind head. Exhale. Gently lower head until light resistance is felt in back, not the ribs—this is a very small motion. Draw lower abdomen in toward spine and gently raise head and arms to starting position.

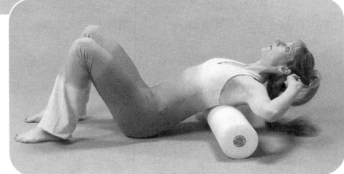

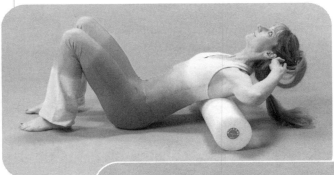

38

Ch4 Stretching

Low Back Stretch

BENEFITS:

To improve range of motion in lower back.

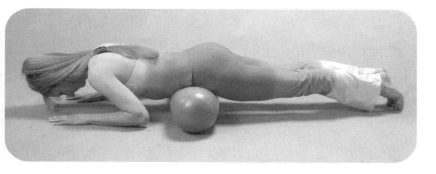

INSTRUCTION: step one

Kneel. Lie on abdomen with roller placed beneath hipbone. Place hands face down on floor with elbows bent.

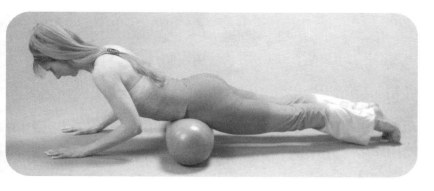

INSTRUCTION: step two

Gently draw lower abdomen toward spine and press up with hands. Maintain a neutral spine in neck and back.

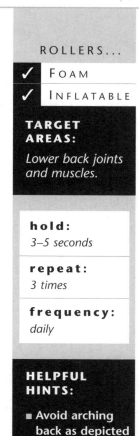

ROLLERS...

✓ FOAM
✓ INFLATABLE

TARGET AREAS:

Lower back joints and muscles.

hold:
3–5 seconds

repeat:
3 times

frequency:
daily

HELPFUL HINTS:

- Avoid arching back as depicted below.
- Neutral spine: A position where back and neck are not arched or flat, they are somewhere in between.

Ch4 Stretching

exercise

7

★☆☆☆☆ **Pelvic Tilts**

ROLLERS...

✓ FOAM

✓ INFLATABLE

It is more comfortable to sit on an inflatable roller.

TARGET AREAS:
Abdominal muscles.

hold:
20 seconds

repeat:
3 times

frequency:
daily

notes

_____

_____

_____

BENEFITS:

This exercise will improve pelvic flexibility and strengthen abdominal muscles making it easier to attain good posture.

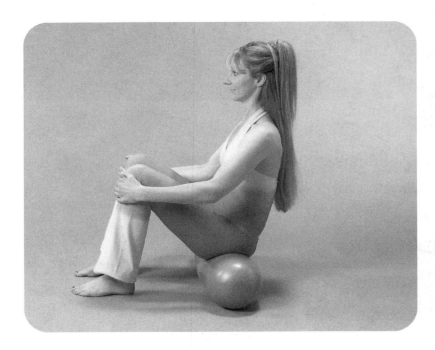

INSTRUCTION: step one

Sit on roller with feet shoulder-width apart and gently place hands on knees. Maintain a neutral spine by drawing lower abdomen toward the spine. Roll roller forward as hips roll backward (round back).

40

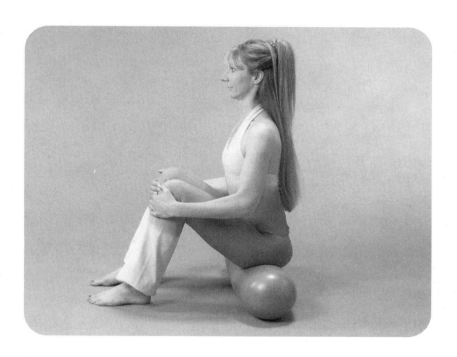

INSTRUCTION: step two

Return to starting position. Roll ball backward as hips roll forward (arched back). Return to starting position.

Ch4 Stretching

8

★★☆☆☆

Hamstring Stretch

ROLLERS...

✓ FOAM

✓ INFLATABLE

It is more comfortable to sit on an inflatable roller.

TARGET AREAS:

Hamstrings

hold:
20 seconds

repeat:
3 times

frequency:
daily

HELPFUL HINTS:

■ Continue to breathe throughout the exercise.

BENEFITS:

To elongate the muscles located in thighs. By improving flexibility in the hamstring muscles (back of thighs) you may prevent or decrease low back pain.

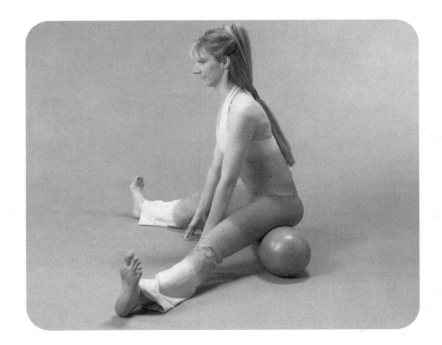

INSTRUCTION:

Sit on roller with legs straight out in front of body. Separate feet as far apart as comfortable. Sit up straight by drawing lower abdomen toward spine.

Core Strength Training © *2006 Caroline Corning Creager 1-800-530-6878*

Trunk Rotation

★ ☆ ☆ ☆ ☆

BENEFITS:

This stretch improves flexibility throughout the spine. Gentle rotation to the spine can help improve circulation to the discs located between the vertebrae (spinal bones).

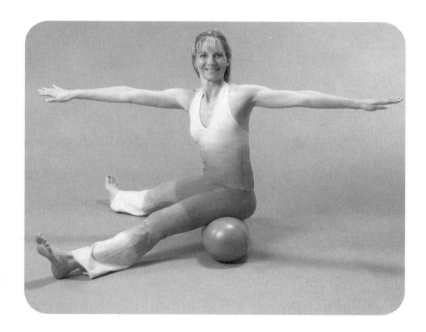

INSTRUCTION:

Sit on roller with legs straight out in front of body. Separate feet as far apart as comfortable. Sit up straight by drawing lower abdomen toward spine. Raise arms, making a 90 degree angle with body. Slowly and gently rotate arms and trunk to the left and then to the right.

ROLLERS...

✓ FOAM

✓ INFLATABLE

It is more comfortable to sit on an inflatable roller.

TARGET AREAS:

Neck and back.

hold:
10 seconds in each direction

repeat:
3 times

frequency:
daily

HELPFUL HINTS:

- The majority of people are able to rotate in one direction further than the other. Focus on rotating the same distance on each side.
- Avoid rounding back.

43

10

★★☆☆☆

Iliotibial Band Massage

ROLLERS...

✓ FOAM

The firm nature of the foam roller is more beneficial for this exercise, however it can also cause more discomfort.

✓ INFLATABLE

Individuals new to this exercise may find the inflatable roller more comfortable.

TARGET AREAS:

Sides of thighs.

hold:
20 seconds

repeat:
3 times

frequency:
daily

BENEFITS:

This exercise will help lengthen the iliotibial band located on the side of the thigh. It may also reduce knee pain. A tight iliotibial band can pull the knee cap (patella) laterally, toward the outer thigh, causing misalignment of the patella. Elongating the iliotibial band can improve patella alignment and therefore eliminate knee pain.

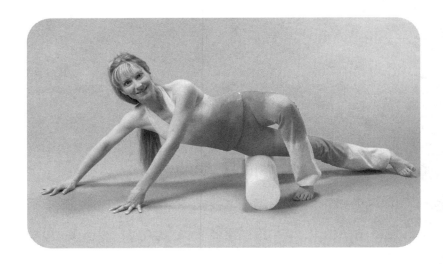

INSTRUCTION: step one

Lie on right side. Place roller under right thigh and place left leg over and in front of right.

Ch4 Stretching

Core Strength Training © 2006 Caroline Corning Creager 1-800-530-6878

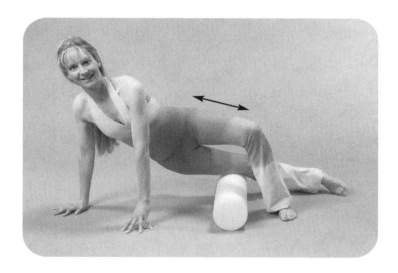

INSTRUCTION: step two

Gently roll roller up and down, from knee to hip. Return to starting position and perform exercise on opposite side.

Piriformis Stretch

ROLLERS...

✓ FOAM
✓ INFLATABLE

TARGET AREAS:

Buttock muscles.

hold:
20 seconds

repeat:
3 times

frequency:
daily

HELPFUL HINTS:

- Avoid raising hips off floor.
- Continue to breathe throughout the exercise.

BENEFITS:

This stretch improves flexibility and circulation in the buttocks.

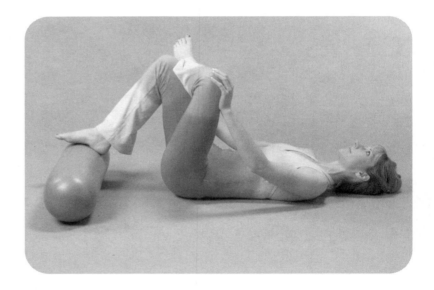

INSTRUCTION:

Lie on back with knees bent. Place right foot on roller and left foot on right knee. Allow left knee to roll out sideways. Draw right foot toward buttock as right hand gently pushes down on left knee. Return to starting position and perform on opposite side.

Core Strength Training © *2006 Caroline Corning Creager 1-800-530-6878*

Prone Quadriceps Stretch

★☆☆☆☆

BENEFITS:

This exercise will elongate the muscles located in the front of the thighs. By improving flexibility in the quadriceps muscles you will improve your standing posture.

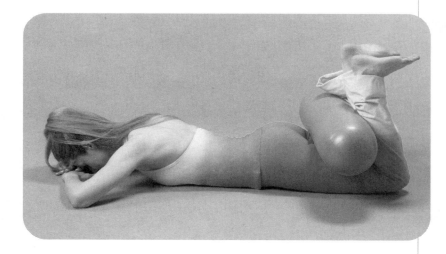

INSTRUCTION:

Lie on abdomen and place roller above knees.
Bend knees and flex toes. Gently squeeze roller with calves.

ROLLERS...

✓ FOAM
✓ INFLATABLE

TARGET AREAS:
Front of thighs.

hold:
20 seconds

repeat:
3 times

frequency:
daily

HELPFUL HINTS:

■ The Prone Quadriceps Stretch requires less balance than the Kneeling Quadriceps Stretch.

■ Avoid raising hips off floor.

■ Continue to breathe throughout the exercise.

Ch4 Stretching

13

★★☆☆☆ **Hip Flexor Stretch**

TARGET AREAS:

Front of hip muscles.

hold:
20 seconds

repeat:
3 times

frequency:
daily

HELPFUL HINTS:

■ Avoid arching or rounding back.

■ Neutral spine: A position where back is not arched or flat, it is somewhere in between.

BENEFITS:

If done incorrectly, sit-ups can cause the hip flexors or front hip muscles to become very tight. This exercise will stretch the hip flexors and improve pelvic flexibility.

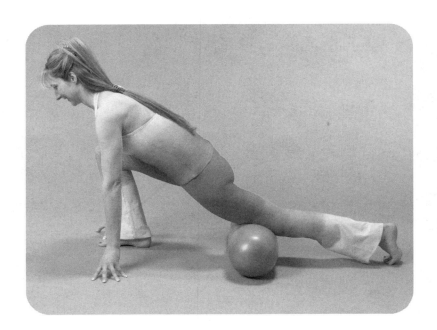

INSTRUCTION:

Kneel. Place roller horizontally on floor behind body. Place left knee on roller and slide back until roller is positioned just above knee. Maintain a neutral spine. Return to starting position and perform exercise on opposite side.

Ch4 Stretching

Hip Flexor & Quadriceps Stretch ★★★☆☆

BENEFITS:

Low back pain and standing with an arch in the low back can cause the hip flexors (deep hip muscles) to become very tight. This exercise will stretch the hip flexors and quadriceps (front thigh) muscles thus improving pelvic flexibility and standing posture.

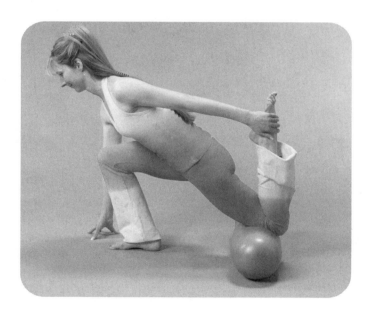

INSTRUCTION:

Kneel. Place roller horizontally on floor behind body. Place left knee on roller and slide back until roller is positioned just above knee. Maintain a neutral spine. Slowly bend left knee and grasp foot with left hand. Return to starting position and perform exercise on opposite side.

ROLLERS...

✓ FOAM
✓ INFLATABLE

It is more comfortable to place the knee on an inflatable roller.

TARGET AREAS:

Front of hip and thigh muscles.

hold:
20 seconds

repeat:
3 times

frequency:
daily

HELPFUL HINTS:

- Avoid arching or rounding back.
- Neutral spine: A position where back is not arched or flat, it is somewhere in between.

Ch4 Stretching

Quadriceps Stretch on Roller

ROLLERS...

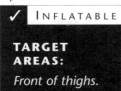 **x** FOAM

*Kneeling on the foam roller is uncomfortable, **HOWEVER**, kneeling on a half roller with flat surface up is a more comfortable option.*

✓ INFLATABLE

TARGET AREAS:

Front of thighs.

hold:
20 seconds

repeat:
3 times

frequency:
daily

HELPFUL HINTS:

■ **Avoid rounding back**

■ **Continue to breathe throughout the exercise.**

BENEFITS:

To elongate the muscles located in the front of the thighs. By improving flexibility in the quadriceps muscles you will improve your posture.

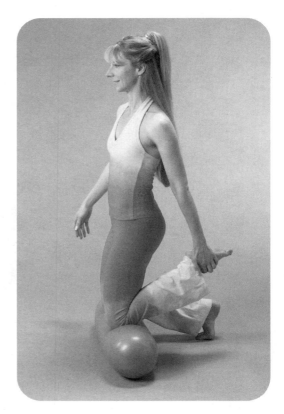

INSTRUCTION:

Kneel on roller. Raise left foot and grasp it with left hand. Maintain a neutral spine position. Lower foot to floor and repeat with opposite side.

Core Strength Training © *2006 Caroline Corning Creager 1-800-530-6878*

Kneeling Quadriceps Stretch ★★★☆☆

BENEFITS:

This variation requires less balance than the Quadriceps Stretch on Roller exercise, but necessitates more balance than the Prone Quadriceps Stretch.

INSTRUCTION:

Kneel on floor with towel roll under knees. Place feet on top of roller. Raise left foot and grasp it with left hand. Maintain a neutral spine position. Hold. Lower foot to roller and repeat with opposite side.

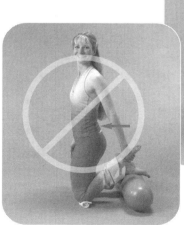

Avoid arching back or bending at waist as depicted at left.

ROLLERS...

✓ FOAM
✓ INFLATABLE

TARGET AREAS:
Front of thighs.

hold:
20 seconds

repeat:
3 times

frequency:
daily

HELPFUL HINTS:

■ The Kneeling Quadriceps Stretch requires more balance than the Prone Quadriceps Stretch. Hence, perform this stretch after you have mastered the Prone Quadriceps Stretch.

Ch4 Stretching

17

★☆☆☆☆

Calf Stretch

ROLLERS...

✓ FOAM
✓ INFLATABLE

TARGET AREAS:
Outer calf muscles.

hold:
20 seconds

repeat:
3 times

frequency:
daily

HELPFUL HINTS:

■ Oftentimes the heel will want to move where the least resistance is, to the left or right of the toes. Maintain heel alignment directly behind the toes.

■ Avoid bending knees.

■ Maintain a neutral spine position.

BENEFITS:

Sitting at a desk throughout the day tightens the calf or gastrocnemius muscles. This exercise stretches the calf muscles and can decrease cramping in them, too.

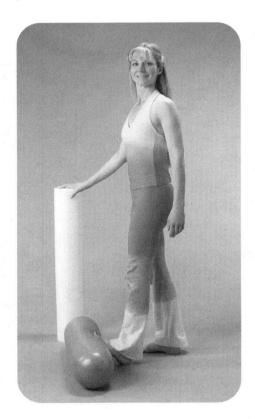

INSTRUCTION:

Place foam roller upright in front of body for balance if needed. Step forward with left foot and place toes on inflatable roller. Flex foot so heel of foot touches floor. Return to starting position and perform on opposite side.

Ch4 Stretching

Soleus Stretch

★☆☆☆☆

BENEFITS:

This exercise improves flexibility in the soleus, or inner calf muscle. Greater flexibility in the soleus muscles will make it easier to climb stairs or walk with a longer stride.

INSTRUCTION:

Place foam roller upright in front of body for balance if needed. Step forward with left foot and place toes on inflatable roller. Flex foot so heel of foot touches floor. Bend knees maintaining knee alignment over feet. Return to starting position and perform on opposite side.

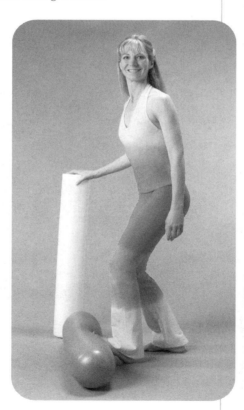

ROLLERS...

✓ FOAM
✓ INFLATABLE

TARGET AREAS:
Inner calf muscles.

hold:
20 seconds

repeat:
3 times

frequency:
daily

HELPFUL HINTS:

■ Oftentimes the heel will want to move where the least resistance is, to the left or right of the toes. Maintain heel alignment directly behind the toes.

■ Maintain a neutral spine position: A position where back is not arched or flat, it is somewhere in between.

Ch4 Stretching

★★★★★

Downward Dog

ROLLERS...

✓ FOAM

✓ INFLATABLE

TARGET AREAS:

Shoulders, back and back of thighs and calves.

hold:
20 seconds

repeat:
3 times

frequency:
daily

HELPFUL HINTS:

■ Avoid rounding back.

■ Continue to breathe throughout the exercise.

■ Neutral spine: A position where back is not arched or flat, it is somewhere in between.

BENEFITS:

To elongate the hamstring muscles, located in the back of the thighs. By improving flexibility in the hamstring muscles you may prevent or decrease low back pain.

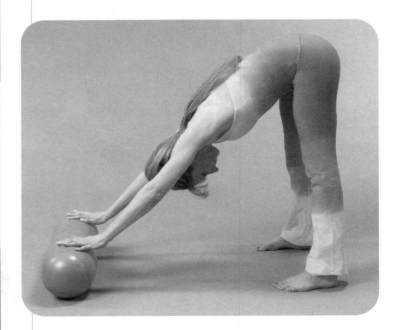

INSTRUCTION:

Stand with feet hip-width apart. Place roller horizontally in front of feet. Lean forward at the hips and place hands on roller. Roll roller in front of body until arms are stretched out straight. Keep head in line with shoulders and maintain a neutral spine. Draw lower abdomen toward spine and return to a standing position.

Ch4 Stretching

Core Strength Training © *2006 Caroline Corning Creager 1-800-530-6878*

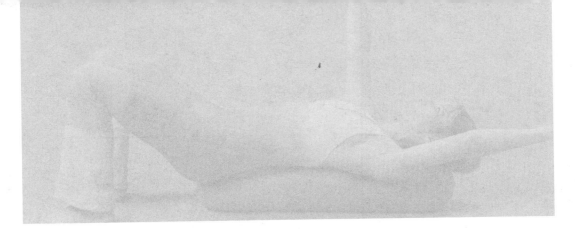

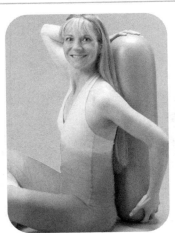

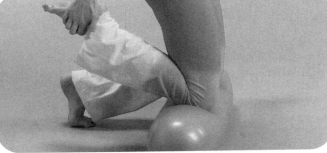

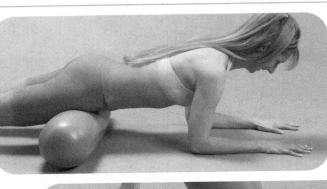

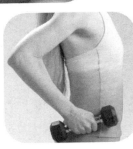

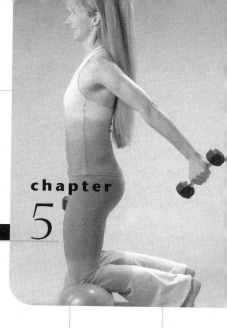

Strengthening Exercise Techniques

The American College of Sports Medicine (ACSM), 1990, recommends that a minimum of 8–10 resistive exercises be performed at least two times per week using major muscle groups.

Each exercise should include a minimum of one set with 8 to 12 repetitions. Roller strengthening exercises are considered resistive exercises, since your body weight is used as the resistance.

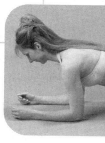

Strengthening exercises should be preceded by a 5-10 minute low-intensity warm-up, 15-20 minutes of stretching exercises, another 15-20 minutes afterwards, and a 5 minute cool down. (Smith, 1994). Warm-up and cool down activities may include a variety of activities — walking, bouncing on the ball while swinging your arms, or pushing your child in a stroller.

Repetitions

How many repetitions (reps), or times, should an exercise be performed? The ACSM recommends you perform each exercise 8 to 12 times. However, remember that the ACSM recommendations are only guidelines.

I frequently recommend less than 6 repetitions for specific exercises throughout the book. I believe many of the roller exercises are more difficult to perform, due to the roller's unstable nature requiring the body to recruit more muscles to perform an exercise, than dumbbell strength exercises. Fewer repetitions at the initiation of an exercise program will also help you focus on your form and quality of motion instead of quantity.

The bottom line is, before you can increase the number of repetitions, the quality of your exercise must be good. When your body begins to fatigue, it causes you to substitute or use incorrect muscles to perform an exercise. For instance, if you are performing the Hip Extension exercise (illustration 5.1) and you are able to perform 6 repetitions before fatigue and on the 7th repetition you begin to arch your back or raise your leg too high (illustration 5.2), then it is time to stop. You would have a 6 repetition maximum (6 RM) for this exercise. Regardless of recommended repetitions in this book, or by the ACSM, you must decide how many repetitions and sets are best for you by following the guidelines established in this book and 'listening' to your body and deciding when it becomes fatigued or begins to substitute muscles incorrectly.

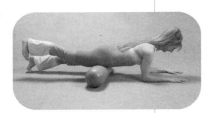

5.1 Hip Extension

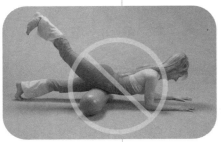

5.2 Hip Extension Raising
Leg <u>Too</u> High

"Most studies have found that RMs that allow for six or fewer repetitions (i.e., low RMs) provide the most strength and power benefits, that weights (roller strengthening exercises) based on 6 RM-12 RM provide moderate strength, power, and endurance gains; and that weights based on RMs of 20 and above provide primarily muscular endurance gains with no strength gain." (Baechle, 1994, pg. 442).

Sets

What is a set? A set is a specific number of repetitions completed without a rest break. If the recommended repetitions for a specific exercise are 8, then you would perform 8 repetitions in each set. When first beginning an exercise program, I recommend you perform one set of each exercise and progress to two and three sets when you are able to maintain good form throughout all repetitions.

Rest

A brief rest period is recommended between each exercise set and between different exercises. This rest period allows your muscles time to recuperate for the next set or exercise. A standard rest period of 30 to 60 seconds (Baechle, 1994) is to be used between sets and exercises in this book, unless otherwise noted. As your fitness level improves, you may begin decreasing the rest period to 15 seconds. The following is a good rule of thumb for deciding when to decrease your rest period: when your heart rate returns to 100 to 110 beats per minute and you are able to maintain good form with a reduced rest period.

Frequency

As stated previously, the ACSM recommends that resistive training be performed at least two times per week. Roller strengthening exercises may be performed in one longer session per day or several brief sessions per day. When performing one star and two star exercises, you may perform them every day. However, when you begin doing three, four, and five star exercises, it is best to alternate days you perform the exercises. For example, strengthen your upper body and abdominal muscles on Monday, Wednesday, and Friday, and strengthen the lower body and back on Tuesday, Thursday, and Saturday.

Sequence of Exercises

Exercise sequence is dependent upon muscle size, which areas of the body are weak, and your exercise goal. Weak or small muscles tend to fatigue more quickly, so they should be placed at the beginning of an exercise regimen. These muscles should be exercised more frequently with a greater number of repetitions. If your goal is to work out in the least amount of time with the greatest benefits, then the following exercise sequencing techniques are of benefit.

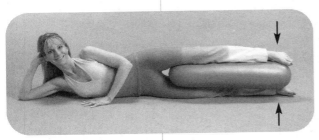

5.3 Inner Thigh Squeeze

Supersetting

Supersetting involves exercising two opposing body parts with a minimal rest break between exercises. Circuit training is a form of superset exercises. For example, you would perform a bicep curl followed by a tricep press. Or, perform an Inner Thigh Squeeze (see illustration 5.3) followed by an Outer Thigh Raise (see illustration 5.4). Supersetting allows opposing muscle groups more time to recuperate than with compound or pre-exhaustion techniques, since there is a greater rest period between exercises for the same muscle groups.

5.4 Outer Thigh Raise

Compound Setting

Compound Setting entails exercising one muscle group with two different exercises in an alternating manner. This mode of exercising is more intense than supersetting. For example, you would perform a sit-up followed by a diagonal sit-up or perform a Sideways Crunch (see illustration 5.5) followed by a Tummy Trimmin' Trunk Curl (see illustration 5.6).

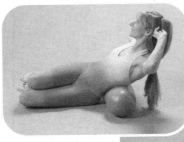

5.5 Sideways Crunch

5.6 Tummy Trimmin' Trunk Curl

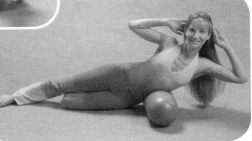

Core Strength Training *© 2006 Caroline Corning Creager 1-800-530-6878*

Pre-exhaustion

Pre-exhaustion is a technique used to focus on strengthening one muscle followed with an exercise that targets many muscles. This mode of exercise is also more intense than supersetting. For example, you would perform a Bicep Curl followed by a Power Clean. Or, perform a Hip Extension (see illustration 5.7) followed by a Standing Plank (see illustration 5.8).

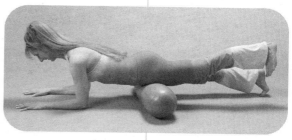

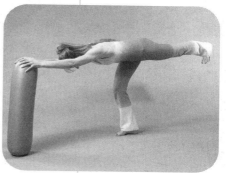

Supersetting, compound setting, and pre-exhaustion techniques require you to be in much better shape than when you perform a few exercises. However, they add variety to the workout, and provide greater strength gains in less time (Baechle, 1994). For ideas on how to implement these techniques, please refer to Mini-Workouts in Chapter VII.

5.7 Hip Extension (top)
5.8 Standing Plank (bottom)

Flow Chart

I have provided a flow chart at the end of the Strengthening Chapter, page 163, so that you may record your progress on the number of sets and repetitions of each exercise completed, along with your daily exercise heart rate. An example is provided on page 163 to show you how to fill out the flow chart correctly. By recording your sets, repetitions, and resting heart rate you can follow your weekly progress at a glance. If you are unfamiliar with taking your pulse to calculate your exercise heart rate, please refer to How to Take Your Pulse on page 199.

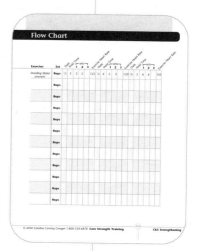

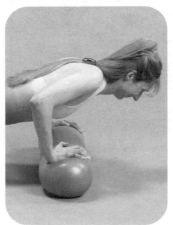

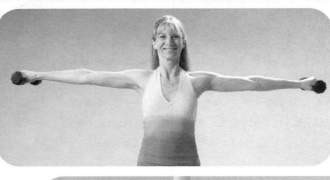

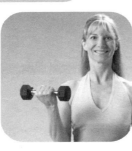

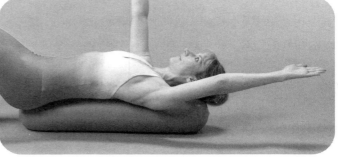

Upper Body Exercises

Body
Exercises

Ch5 Strengthening

★☆☆☆☆

Unilateral Bicep Curl

ROLLERS...

✓ FOAM

*It may be uncomfortable to kneel on the full foam roller. **HOWEVER**, kneeling on a half roller with flat surface up is a comfortable option.*

✓ INFLATABLE

TARGET AREAS:

Front arm and 'core' muscles.

hold:
2 seconds

repeat:
1–3 set(s), 8–12 reps each side

frequency:
2–3 times per week

HELPFUL HINTS:

■ Avoid arching back. Men tend to have less flexibility in their quadriceps (front thigh muscles) and hip muscles and therefore may have more difficulty maintaining a neutral spine in the kneeling position.

BENEFITS:

The bicep muscle, located in the front of the arm, is a strong muscle. Kneeling on a roller using hand weights, as depicted, will not only improve your balance, but increase strength in the bicep muscle and in your 'core' muscles.

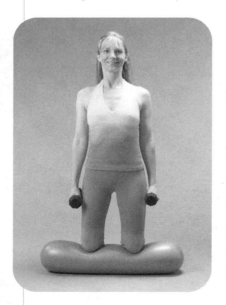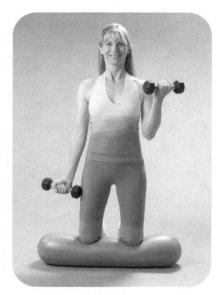

INSTRUCTION:

Grasp a pair of dumbbells and kneel with roller positioned underneath knees. Allow arms to hang straight down below shoulders. Maintain a neutral neck and spine position (A position where neck and back are not arched or flat, but somewhere in between). Gently draw lower abdomen toward spine and curl weight upward rotating palm up. Curl as high as possible without moving upper arm forward. Hold. Return to starting position. Repeat with opposite side.

Bilateral Bicep Curl

VARIATION

BENEFITS:

It is best to challenge your muscles with different exercise options, so switch between the Unilateral and Bilateral Bicep Curls.

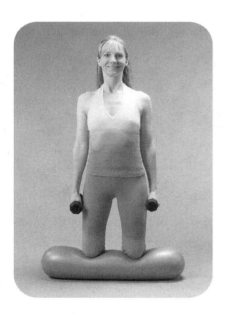
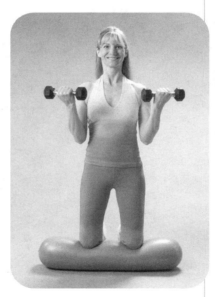

INSTRUCTION:

Follow directions from Exercise 1, Unilateral Bicep Curl, however bend both arms simultaneously.

ROLLERS...

✓ FOAM

It may be uncomfortable to kneel on the full foam roller. **HOWEVER,** *kneeling on a half roller with flat surface up is a comfortable option.*

✓ INFLATABLE

TARGET AREAS:

Front arm and 'core' muscles.

hold:
2 seconds

repeat:
1–3 sets, 8–12 reps

frequency:
2–3 times per week

HELPFUL HINTS:

- Keep neck muscles relaxed.
- Avoid arching back.

Ch5 Strengthening

3

exercise

★★☆☆☆

Unilateral Tricep Extension

ROLLERS...

✓ FOAM

It may be uncomfortable to kneel on the full foam roller. **HOWEVER,** *kneeling on a half roller with flat surface up is a comfortable option.*

✓ INFLATABLE

TARGET AREAS:

Front arm and 'core' muscles.

hold:
2 seconds

repeat:
1–3 set(s), 8–12 reps each side

frequency:
2–3 times per week

HELPFUL HINTS:

■ Avoid arching back. Men tend to have less flexibility in their quadriceps (front thigh muscles and) and hip muscles and therefore may have more difficulty maintaining a neutral spine in the kneeling position.

BENEFITS:

The tricep muscle, located in the back of the arm, is typically weaker than the bicep muscle. Kneeling on a roller using hand weights, as depicted, will not only improve your balance but increase strength in the tricep muscle and in your 'core' muscles.

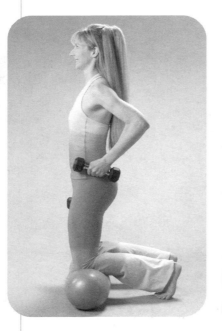
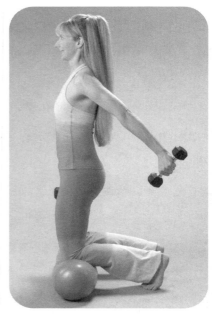

INSTRUCTION:

Grasp a pair of dumbbells and kneel with roller positioned underneath knees. Bend elbow, placing hand close to hip and in alignment with shoulder. Maintain a neutral neck and spine position (A position where neck and back are not arched or flat, but somewhere in between). Gently draw lower abdomen toward spine and straighten left arm rotating thumb down. Hold. Return to starting position. Repeat with opposite side.

66

Ch5 Strengthening

Bilateral Tricep Extension

★★★☆☆

VARIATION

BENEFITS:

The dynamic nature of the roller and your change in center of gravity (from moving both arms backward at the same time) makes this exercise more difficult than the Unilateral Tricep Extension. It is best to challenge your muscles with different exercise options, so switch between the Unilateral and Bilateral Tricep Extensions.

ROLLERS...

✓ FOAM

*It may be uncomfortable to kneel on the full foam roller. **HOWEVER**, kneeling on a half roller with flat surface up is a comfortable option.*

✓ INFLATABLE

TARGET AREAS:

Back arm and 'core' muscles.

hold:
2 seconds

repeat:
1–3 sets, 8–12 reps

frequency:
2–3 times per week

HELPFUL HINTS:

- Keep neck muscles relaxed.
- Avoid arching back.

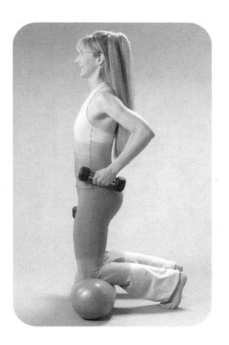
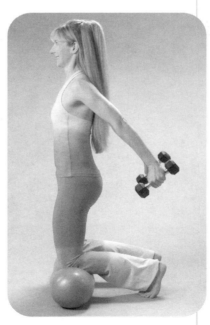

INSTRUCTION:

Follow directions from Exercise 3, Unilateral Tricep Extension, however straighten both arms, rotating thumbs down.

67

★★☆☆☆

Tricep Press

ROLLERS...

✓ FOAM

✓ INFLATABLE

TARGET AREAS:

Back of arm muscles.

hold:
5–15 seconds

repeat:
1–3 sets, 8–12 reps

frequency:
2–3 times per week

HELPFUL HINTS:

- Avoid winging elbow away from head. By maintaining an elbow position close to your head. You will target the tricep muscles.
- Keep neck muscles relaxed.
- Avoid tucking or tipping chin back.
- Avoid arching back.

BENEFITS:

"Jiggle, jiggle" is what can happen to the back of the arm when you wave your hand. The tricep muscle located beneath 'the jiggle' is often very weak, especially with women. By adding muscle bulk to the back of the arm, you will decrease the unwanted wiggle in your arm.

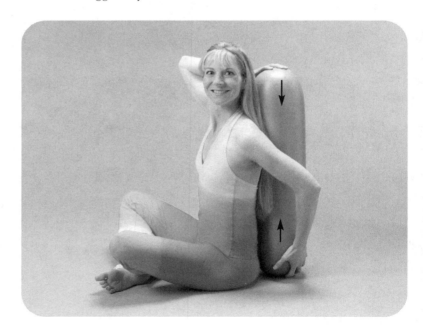

INSTRUCTION:

Sit with roller positioned upright behind back. Reach right hand behind head and place on top of roller. Place left fingers underneath roller. Press right and left hands together into roller. Return to starting position. Repeat with opposite side.

Unilateral Shoulder Flexion ★★★☆☆

BENEFITS:

Kneeling on a roller using hand weights, as depicted, will not only improve your balance but increase strength in the shoulder and 'core' muscles.

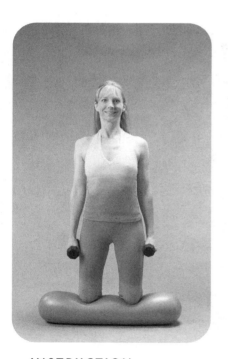 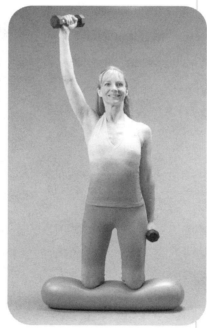

INSTRUCTION:

Grasp a pair of dumbbells and kneel with roller positioned underneath knees. Allow arms to hang straight down below shoulders. Keep eyes level and maintain a neutral neck and spine position (A position where neck and back are not arched or flat, but somewhere in between). Gently draw lower abdomen toward spine and raise right arm overhead. Hold. Return to starting position. Repeat with opposite arm.

ROLLERS...

✓ FOAM

It may be uncomfortable to kneel on the full foam roller. **HOWEVER,** *kneeling on a half roller with flat surface up is a comfortable option.*

✓ INFLATABLE

TARGET AREAS:

Front of shoulder and 'core' muscles.

hold:
2 seconds

repeat:
1–3 sets, 8–12 reps each side

frequency:
2–3 times per week

HELPFUL HINTS:

■ Keep neck muscles relaxed.
■ Avoid arching back.

Ch5 Strengthening

Bilateral Shoulder Flexion

ROLLERS...

✓ FOAM

It may be uncomfortable to kneel on the full foam roller. **HOWEVER,** *kneeling on a half roller with flat surface up is a comfortable option.*

✓ INFLATABLE

TARGET AREAS:

Front of shoulder and 'core' muscles.

hold:
2 seconds

repeat:
1–3 set(s), 6–12 reps

frequency:
2–3 times per week

HELPFUL HINTS:

■ Avoid arching back. Men tend to have less flexibility in their quadriceps (front thigh muscles) and hip muscles and therefore may have more difficulty maintaining a neutral spine in the kneeling position.

BENEFITS:

Due to the dynamic nature of the roller, raising both arms at the same time can make this exercise more difficult than the Unilateral Shoulder Flexion. It is best to challenge your muscles with different exercise options, so switch between the Unilateral and Bilateral Shoulder Flexion exercises.

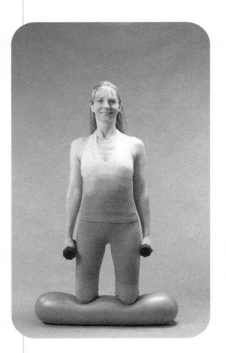 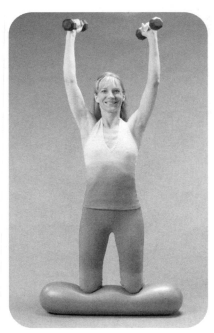

INSTRUCTION:

Follow directions from Exercise 6, Unilateral Shoulder Flexion, however, raise both arms overhead.

Ch5 Strengthening

Core Strength Training © *2006 Caroline Corning Creager 1-800-530-6878*

Unilateral Shoulder Extension ★★☆☆☆

BENEFITS:

The shoulder extension exercise strengthens muscles on the backside of the shoulder region and stretches the muscles on the front of the shoulder. It is best to challenge your muscles with different exercise options, so switch between the Unilateral and Bilateral Shoulder Extensions.

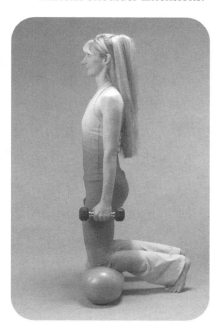

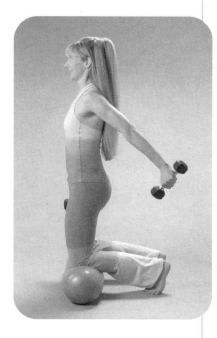

INSTRUCTION:

Grasp a pair of dumbbells and kneel with roller positioned underneath knees. Position straight arms next to body. Keep eyes level and maintain a neutral neck and spine position. Gently draw lower abdomen toward spine and raise left arm behind back with thumb toward floor. Hold. Return to starting position. Repeat with opposite side.

ROLLERS...

✓ FOAM

It may be uncomfortable to kneel on the full foam roller. **HOWEVER,** *kneeling on a half roller with flat surface up is a comfortable option.*

✓ INFLATABLE

TARGET AREAS:
Front and back of shoulder 'core' muscles.

hold:
2 seconds

repeat:
1–3 set(s), 8–12 reps

frequency:
2–3 times per week

HELPFUL HINTS:

- **Keep neck muscles relaxed.**
- **Avoid arching back.**

71

exercise

9

★ ★ ☆ ☆ ☆

Bilateral Shoulder Extension

ROLLERS...

✓ FOAM

*It may be uncomfortable to kneel on the full foam roller. **HOWEVER**, kneeling on a half roller with flat surface up is a comfortable option.*

✓ INFLATABLE

TARGET AREAS:

Back of shoulder & 'core' muscles.

hold:
2 seconds

repeat:
1–3 set(s), 8–12 reps

frequency:
2–3 times per week

HELPFUL HINTS:

■ Avoid arching back. Men tend to have less flexibility in their quadriceps (front thigh muscles) and hip muscles and therefore may have more difficulty maintaining a neutral spine in the kneeling position.

BENEFITS:

The Bilateral Shoulder Extension exercise not only strengthens muscles on the backside of the shoulder, it will also challenge your balance by changing your center of gravity. It is best to challenge your muscles with different exercise options, so switch between the Unilateral and Bilateral Shoulder Extensions.

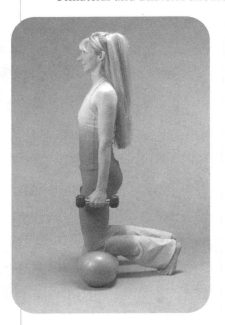
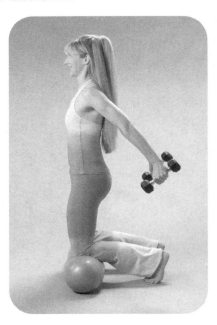

INSTRUCTION:

Grasp a pair of dumbbells and kneel with roller positioned underneath knees. Position straight arms next to body. Keep eyes level and maintain a neutral neck and spine position. Gently draw lower abdomen toward spine and raise both arms behind back with thumbs toward floor. Hold. Return to starting position.

Ch5 Strengthening

Shoulder Flexion & Extension

BENEFITS:

Kneeling on a roller using hand weights, as depicted, will not only improve your balance, but also increase strength in the shoulder muscles and in your "core muscles". This exercise promotes reciprocal arm movement as with walking or running.

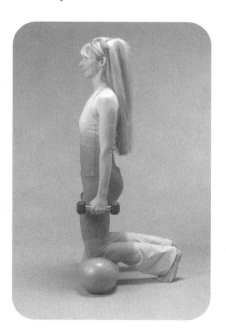

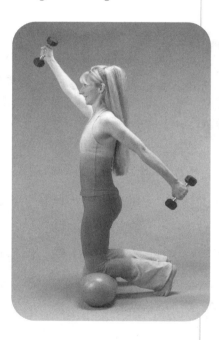

INSTRUCTION:

Grasp a pair of dumbbells and kneel with roller positioned underneath knees. Allow arms to hang straight down below shoulders. Keep eyes level and maintain a neutral neck and spine position. Gently draw lower abdomen toward spine. Raise right arm in front of body and extend left arm behind back. Hold. Return to starting position. Repeat with opposite arm.

ROLLERS...

✓ FOAM

It may be uncomfortable to kneel on the full foam roller. **HOWEVER,** *kneeling on a half roller with flat surface up is a comfortable option.*

✓ INFLATABLE

TARGET AREAS:

Front & back of shoulders & 'core' muscles.

hold:
2 seconds

repeat:
1–3 set(s), 8–12 reps

frequency:
2–3 times per week

HELPFUL HINTS:

■ Keep neck muscles relaxed.
■ Avoid arching back.

Ch5 Strengthening

Supraspinatus Raise

ROLLERS...

✓ FOAM

It may be uncomfortable to kneel on the full foam roller. **HOWEVER,** *kneeling on a half roller with flat surface up is a comfortable option.*

✓ INFLATABLE

TARGET AREAS:

Back of shoulder and 'core' muscles.

hold:
2 seconds

repeat:
1–3 set(s), 8–12 reps each side

frequency:
2–3 times per week

HELPFUL HINTS:

■ Avoid arching back. Men tend to have less flexibility in their quadriceps (front thigh muscles) and hip muscles and therefore may have more difficulty maintaining a neutral spine in the kneeling position.

BENEFITS:

The supraspinatus muscle is one of the shoulder muscles that make up the rotator cuff. It is also the most common rotator cuff muscle to tear with activity. By strengthening the supraspinatus muscle with this exercise, you will help prevent injuries to it in the future.

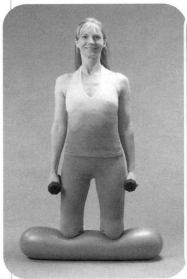 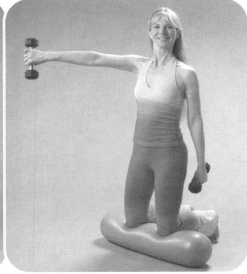

INSTRUCTION:

Grasp a pair of dumbbells and kneel with roller positioned underneath knees. Allow arms to hang straight down aligning below shoulders. Keep eyes level and maintain a neutral neck and spine position. Gently draw lower abdomen toward spine. Rotate thumb toward leg and raise right arm up at a 45 degree angle from front of body, to shoulder height. Hold. Return to starting position. Repeat with opposite arm.

Ch5 Strengthening

Shoulder External Rotation

★★☆☆☆

BENEFITS:

Kneeling on a roller using hand weights, as depicted, will not only improve your balance but also increase strength in the teres minor and infraspinatus muscles, rotator cuff muscles, and in your 'core' muscles.

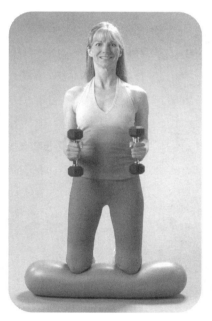 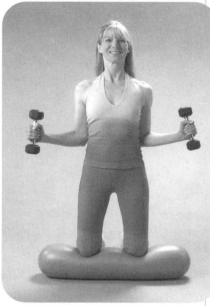

INSTRUCTION:

Grasp a pair of dumbbells and kneel with roller positioned underneath knees. Keep eyes level and maintain a neutral neck and spine position. Gently draw lower abdomen toward spine. Bend elbows, placing elbows close to hips and in alignment with shoulders. Rotate arms out toward side of body, keeping elbows next to body. Hold. Return to starting position.

ROLLERS...

✓ FOAM

It may be uncomfortable to kneel on the full foam roller. **HOWEVER,** *kneeling on a half roller with flat surface up is a comfortable option.*

✓ INFLATABLE

TARGET AREAS:

Back of shoulder and 'core' muscles.

hold:
2 seconds

repeat:
1–3 set(s), 8–12 reps

frequency:
3–4 times per week

HELPFUL HINTS:

- Keep neck muscles relaxed.
- Avoid arching back.

75

Shoulder Circles

✓ FOAM

*It may be uncomfortable to kneel on the full foam roller. **HOWEVER,** kneeling on a half roller with flat surface up is a comfortable option.*

✓ INFLATABLE

TARGET AREAS:

Shoulder and 'core' muscles.

hold:
2 seconds

repeat:
*1–3 set(s),
8–12 reps*

frequency:
2–3 times per week

HELPFUL HINTS:

- Keep neck muscles relaxed.
- Avoid arching back.

BENEFITS:

The Shoulder Circle Exercise will help relieve tension in the shoulders, strengthen shoulder muscles, and improve 'core' strength by challenging your balance.

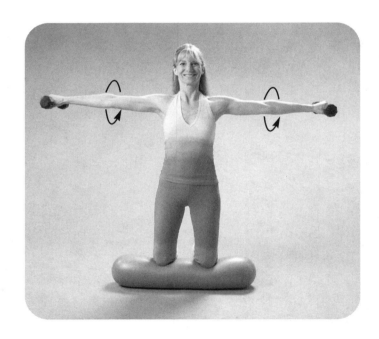

INSTRUCTION:

Grasp a pair of dumbbells and kneel with roller positioned underneath knees. Allow arms to hang straight down aligning below shoulders. Keep eyes level and maintain a neutral neck and spine position. Gently draw lower abdomen toward spine and raise arms away from sides to 90 degrees. Hold. Make small arm circles forward. Return to starting position. Repeat exercise performing small arm circles backward.

Ch5 Strengthening

Shoulder Abduction

★★☆☆☆

BENEFITS:

Men and women often want to make their waist look smaller. By strengthening or bulking up the middle fibers of the deltoid muscle, the side shoulder muscle, you can accomplish just this. When your shoulders are broader it gives the appearance that your waist is smaller. Kneeling on a roller using hand weights, as depicted, will not only improve your balance but increase strength in the deltoid muscle and in your 'core' muscles.

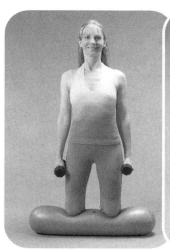 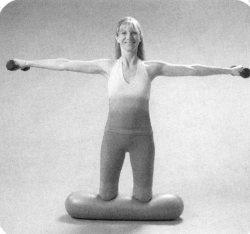

INSTRUCTION:

Grasp a pair of dumbbells and kneel with roller positioned underneath knees. Allow arms to hang straight down below shoulders. Keep eyes level and maintain a neutral neck and spine position. Gently draw lower abdomen toward spine and raise arms away from sides to 90 degrees. Hold. Return to starting position. Repeat.

ROLLERS...

✓ FOAM

It may be uncomfortable to kneel on the full foam roller. **HOWEVER,** *kneeling on a half roller with flat surface up is a comfortable option.*

✓ INFLATABLE

TARGET AREAS:

Side shoulder and 'core' muscles.

hold:
2 seconds

repeat:
1–3 set(s), 8–12 reps

frequency:
2–3 times per week

HELPFUL HINTS:

■ Keep neck muscles relaxed.
■ Avoid arching back.

Ch5 Strengthening

Shoulder Abduction to Overhead

ROLLERS...

✓ **FOAM**

It may be uncomfortable to kneel on the full foam roller. **HOWEVER,** *kneeling on a half roller with flat surface up is a comfortable option.*

✓ **INFLATABLE**

TARGET AREAS:

Front of shoulder 'core' muscles.

hold:
2 seconds

repeat:
1–3 set(s),
6–10 reps

frequency:
3–4 times per week

HELPFUL HINTS:

- Keep neck muscles relaxed.
- Avoid arching back.
- Discontinue exercise if you experience pain.

BENEFITS:

This exercise will strengthen your shoulder muscles at the end of their range. If you experience a pinching sensation in your shoulder with this exercise – only raise your arm as far as you can before you feel the pinching sensation or discontinue exercise.

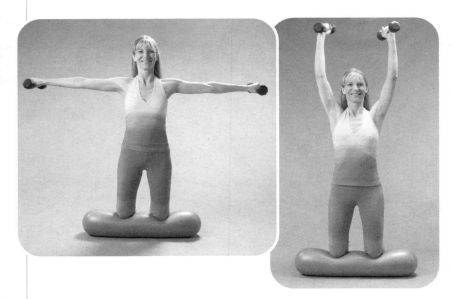

INSTRUCTION:

Follow directions from Exercise 14, Shoulder Abduction. However, after raising both arms away from sides to 90 degrees, rotate palms up and arms overhead.

Ch5 Strengthening

Core Strength Training *© 2006 Caroline Corning Creager 1-800-530-6878*

Supine Position on Roller

★☆☆☆☆

BENEFITS:

This exercise will help strengthen neck and back muscles in an optimal position to prevent injury (during work, exercise, or play.)

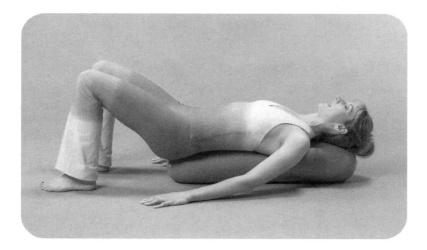

INSTRUCTION:

Lie on side with knees bent. Roll back onto roller with feet flat on floor and arms relaxed down by sides of body. Maintain a natural curve in back and neck or neutral spine position (a position where back and neck are not arched or flat, but somewhere in between).

ROLLERS...

✓ FOAM
✓ INFLATABLE

TARGET AREAS:

Back and neck muscles.

hold:
5–15 seconds

repeat:
*1–3 set(s),
5–12 reps*

frequency:
2–3 times per week

HELPFUL HINTS:

- Please see *Cervical Stabilization* (page 17) and *Pelvic Stabilization* (page 91) for alternate supine roller positions.
- Keep neck muscles relaxed.
- Avoid tucking or tipping chin back.

79

Ch5 Strengthening

17

★★☆☆☆

Cervical Stabilization

ROLLERS...

✓ FOAM

✓ INFLATABLE

TARGET AREAS:
Back and neck muscles.

hold:
5–15 seconds

repeat:
3 reps

frequency:
2–3 times per week

HELPFUL HINTS:

■ Please see *Supine Position on Roller and Pelvic Stabilization* (pages 79, 91) for alternate supine roller positions.

■ Avoid arching or flattening back.

■ Keep neck muscles relaxed.

■ Avoid tucking or tipping chin back.

BENEFITS:

This exercise will help strengthen neck muscles in an optimal position to prevent injury during work, exercise, or play. Placing a ball* under the head, instead of the roller, makes this exercise more difficult. However, this position may be more comfortable for tall people.

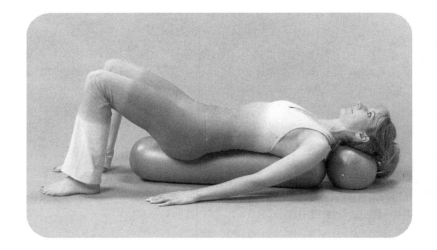

INSTRUCTION:

Lie on side with knees bent. Roll back onto roller with feet flat on floor. Place small ball* under head and arms relaxed down by sides of body. Maintain a natural curve in back and neck or neutral spine position (a position where back and neck are not arched or flat, but somewhere in between) by drawing lower abdomen toward spine.

* The small ball, as depicted in photo, can be purchased from *Orthopedic Physical Therapy Products* by calling 800-367-7393.

Supine Shoulder Flexion/Extension ★☆☆☆☆

BENEFITS:

The latisimus dorsi, a large back muscle, is often very tight. This exercise when performed correctly—raising your arm as high as you can without arching the back—will help lengthen the latisimus dorsi. The core muscles will also be engaged when you raise your arm overhead and maintain your balance on the roller.

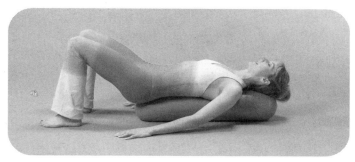

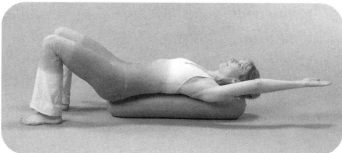

INSTRUCTION:

Lie on side with knees bent. Roll back onto roller with feet flat on floor and arms relaxed down by sides of body. Maintain a natural curve in back and neck or neutral spine position (by drawing lower abdomen toward spine). Raise left arm overhead. Lower arm to starting position. Repeat with opposite side.

ROLLERS...

✓ FOAM
✓ INFLATABLE

TARGET AREAS:

Shoulder, arm, back and neck muscles.

hold:
3 seconds

repeat:
1–3 set(s), 8–12 reps each side

frequency:
2–3 times per week

HELPFUL HINTS:

■ Please see *Cervical and Pelvic Stabilization* (pages 80, 91) for alternate supine roller positions.
■ Avoid arching or flattening back.
■ Keep neck muscles relaxed.
■ Avoid tucking or tipping chin back.

Ch5 Strengthening

Supine Shoulder Pulses

ROLLERS...

✓ FOAM

✓ INFLATABLE

TARGET AREAS:

Arm, neck, shoulder, and trunk muscles.

hold:
3 seconds

repeat:
1–3 set(s), 8–12 reps

frequency:
2–3 times per week

HELPFUL HINTS:

- Please see *Cervical and Pelvic Stabilization* (pages 80, 91) for alternate supine roller positions.

- Avoid arching or flattening back.

- Keep neck muscles relaxed.

- Avoid tucking or tipping chin back.

BENEFITS:

Shoulder pulses and half pulses strengthen the shoulder complex, neck, and core muscles. These exercises also improve balance and coordination.

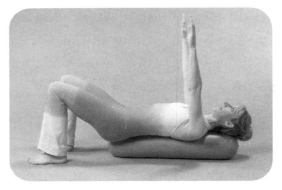

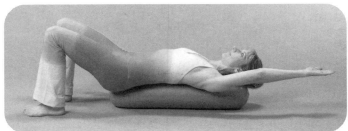

INSTRUCTION:

Lie on side with knees bent. Roll back onto roller with feet flat on floor and arms relaxed down by sides of body. Gently draw lower abdomen toward spine and raise both arms to 90 degrees. Rapidly raise right arm overhead and lower left arm to floor towards feet and switch directions—sustaining a steady position on the roller. Maintain a natural curve in back and neck during exercise.

Ch5 Strengthening

Core Strength Training © *2006 Caroline Corning Creager 1-800-530-6878*

Supine Shoulder Half Pulses ★☆☆☆☆

BENEFITS:

This exercise improves balance, coordination and strengthens upper body and neck.

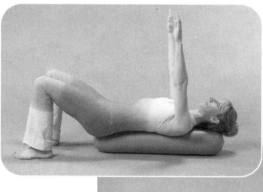

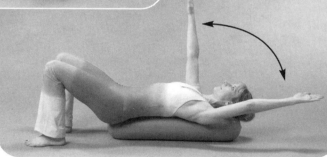

INSTRUCTION:

Lie on side with knees bent. Roll back onto roller with feet flat on floor and arms relaxed down by sides of body. Gently draw lower abdomen toward spine and raise both arms to 90 degrees. Rapidly raise right arm overhead and switch directions, lowering right arm to 90 degrees and raising left arm overhead. Sustaining a steady position and a neutral spine position (a position where back and neck are not arched or flat, but somewhere in between) on roller throughout exercise.

ROLLERS...

✓ FOAM

✓ INFLATABLE

TARGET AREAS:

Arm, neck, shoulder, and trunk muscles.

hold:
1 second

repeat:
1–3 set(s), 8–12 reps

frequency:
2–3 times per week

HELPFUL HINTS:

■ Please see *Cervical and Pelvic Stabilization* (pages 80, 91) for alternate supine roller positions.

■ Avoid arching or flattening back.

■ Keep neck muscles relaxed.

■ Avoid tucking or tipping chin back.

Ch5 Strengthening

21

★★☆☆☆

Lower Trapezius Press

ROLLERS...

✓ FOAM

✓ INFLATABLE

TARGET AREAS:

Mid-back and shoulder blade muscles.

hold:
5–15 seconds

repeat:
*1–3 sets,
8–12 reps each side*

frequency:
2–3 times per week

HELPFUL HINTS:

■ Keep neck muscles relaxed.

■ Avoid tucking or tipping chin back.

■ Avoid arching back.

BENEFITS:

The mid-back muscles are typically very weak, especially as we age. This exercise helps strengthen the muscles between the shoulder blades.

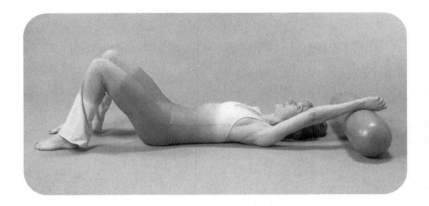

INSTRUCTION: step one

Lie on back with knees bent. Raise left arm overhead and position roller underneath the wrist. Rotate hand so thumb is pointing toward floor.

INSTRUCTION: step two

Press wrist into roller. Return to starting position. Repeat with opposite arm.

Push-Up on Roller–Beginner ★★★☆☆

BENEFITS:

This exercise works the abdomen against gravity, strengthens core muscles, chest, triceps (back of arms), and muscles surrounding the shoulder blades. This exercise challenges your balance and is more difficult than a traditional modified push-up.

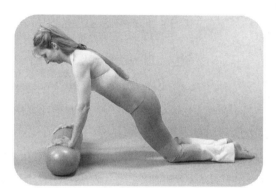

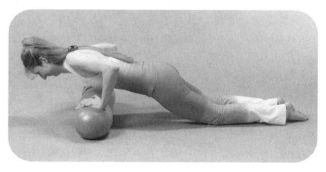

INSTRUCTION:

Kneel. Place roller on floor in front of body. Lean forward so arms are extended out straight, hands are on top of roller shoulder-width apart, and body is in a modified push-up position (knees on floor.) Gently draw lower abdomen toward spine and maintain a neutral spine (a position where back and neck are not arched or flat, but somewhere in between). Slowly lower body down toward roller. Return to modified push-up position.

ROLLERS...

✓ FOAM
✓ INFLATABLE

TARGET AREAS:

Arm, chest, shoulder and trunk muscles.

hold:
2 seconds

repeat:
1–3 set(s), 3–8 reps

frequency:
2–3 times per week

HELPFUL HINTS:

- Avoid hyper-extending elbows by keeping a slight bend in them.
- Avoid arching or rounding back.
- Avoid tucking or tipping chin back.

85

23

★★★★★

Push-Up on Roller–Advanced

ROLLERS...

✓ FOAM

✓ INFLATABLE

TARGET AREAS:

Arm, chest, shoulder and trunk muscles.

hold:
2 seconds

repeat:
1–3 set(s), 3–8 reps

frequency:
2–3 times per week

HELPFUL HINTS:

■ Avoid hyper-extending elbows by keeping a slight bend in them.

■ Avoid arching or rounding back.

■ Avoid tucking or tipping chin back.

BENEFITS:

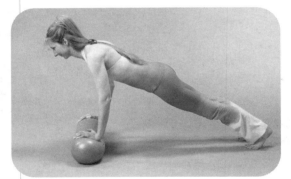

This exercise works the abdomen against gravity, strengthens core muscles, chest, triceps (back of arms), and muscles surrounding the shoulder blades. It challenges your balance and is more difficult than a traditional push-up. This exercise can cause discomfort in the wrist. If you experience wrist pain or discomfort, try performing a push-up with hands on the floor as illustrated on the next page.

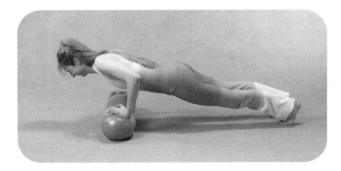

INSTRUCTION:

Kneel. Place roller on floor at right angle to body. Lean forward so arms are extended out straight and hands are on top of roller shoulder-width apart. Gently draw lower abdomen toward spine and maintain a neutral spine. Straighten legs so body is in a push-up position. Slowly lower body down toward roller. Return to a push-up position.

Push-Up

★★★★☆

BENEFITS:

This exercise works the abdomen against gravity, strengthens core muscles, chest, triceps (back of arms), and muscles surrounding shoulder blades. It challenges your balance and is more difficult than a traditional push-up. This exercise can cause discomfort in the wrist. If you experience wrist pain or discomfort, try performing a push-up with hands in a fist, so knuckles touch the floor and wrists are straight.

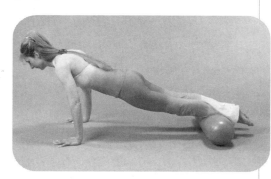

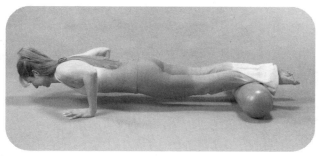

INSTRUCTION:

Kneel and position roller beneath ankles. Lean forward so arms are extended out straight and hands are shoulder-width apart. Gently draw lower abdomen toward spine and maintain a neutral spine (a position where back and neck are not arched or flat, but somewhere in between). Straighten legs and assume a push-up position. Slowly lower body down toward floor. Return to push-up position.

ROLLERS...

✓ FOAM

✓ INFLATABLE

TARGET AREAS:

Arm, chest, shoulder and trunk muscles.

hold:
2 seconds

repeat:
1–3 set(s), 3–8 reps

frequency:
2–3 times per week

HELPFUL HINTS:

■ Avoid hyper-extending elbows by keeping a slight bend in them.

■ Avoid arching or rounding back.

■ Avoid tucking or tipping chin back.

87

Ch5 Strengthening

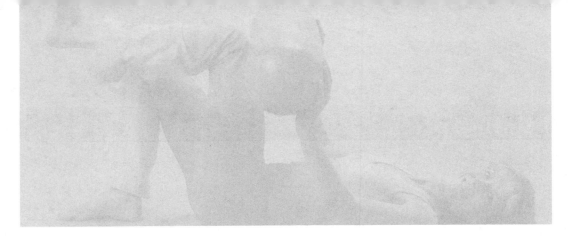

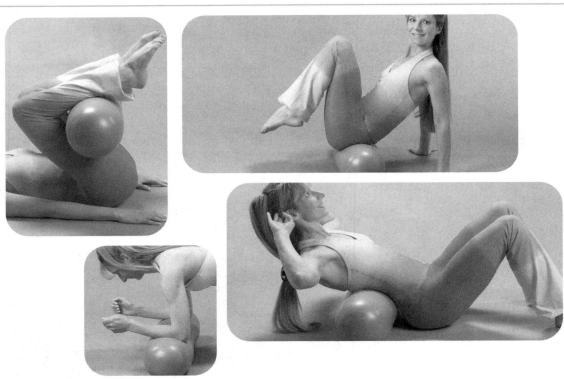

Core Body Exercises

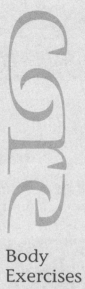

Body
Exercises

25

★☆☆☆☆

Pelvic Tilt

ROLLERS...

✓ FOAM
✓ INFLATABLE

TARGET AREAS:
Abdominal muscles.

hold:
3 seconds

repeat:
1–3 set(s), 6–12 reps

frequency:
2–3 times per week

HELPFUL HINTS:

- This exercise can be used as both a strengthening exercise for the abdomen and a stretching exercise for abdomen and lower back.

BENEFITS:

This exercise will strengthen abdominal muscles and help improve standing posture. If you have an exaggerated arch in your low back in a standing position, focus more on rounding your back as in photo on left. If you tend to have a flat back, concentrate on arching your back as in photo on right.

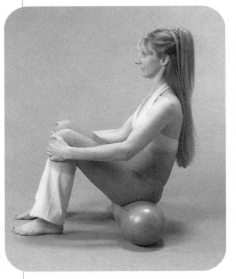 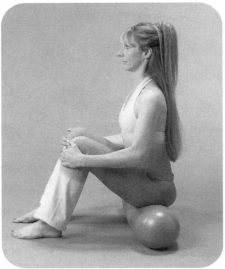

INSTRUCTION:

Sit on roller with knees bent and hip-width apart. Maintain a neutral spine (a position where back is not arched or flat, it is somewhere in between) by drawing lower abdomen toward spine. Push roller forward as hips roll backward (round back). Hold. Push roller backward as hips roll forward (arched back).

Ch5 Strengthening

Pelvic Stabilization

★☆☆☆☆

BENEFITS:

This exercise strengthens pelvic muscles in an optimal position to avoid injury during work, exercise, or play. Placing a ball* under the pelvis, instead of the roller, makes this exercise more difficult. However, this position may be more comfortable for tall people.

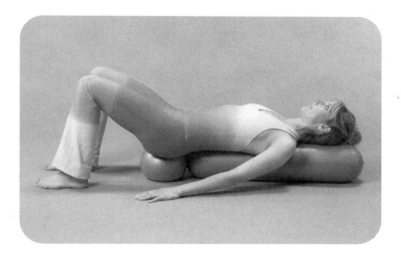

INSTRUCTION:

Lie on side with knees bent. Roll back onto roller with feet flat on floor. Place small ball under pelvis and arms relaxed down by sides of body. Maintain a natural curve in back and neck or neutral spine position (a position where back is not arched or flat, it is somewhere in between) by drawing lower abdomen toward spine.

* The small ball, as depicted in photo, can be purchased from *Orthopedic Physical Therapy Products* by calling 800-367-7393.

ROLLERS...

✓ FOAM
✓ INFLATABLE

TARGET AREAS:

Pelvic, back and neck muscles.

hold:
5–15 seconds

repeat:
1–3 set(s), 5–15 reps

frequency:
2–3 times per week

HELPFUL HINTS:

■ Please see *Supine Position on Roller* and *Cervical Stabilization* (pages 79, 80) for alternate supine roller positions.

■ Avoid arching or flattening back.

■ Keep neck muscles relaxed.

■ Avoid tucking or tipping chin back.

91

Ch5 Strengthening

Abdominal Bracing

ROLLERS...

✓ FOAM
✓ INFLATABLE

TARGET AREAS:
Abdominal and hip muscles.

hold:
3 seconds

repeat:
1–2 set(s), 6–12 reps each leg

frequency:
2–3 times per week

HELPFUL HINTS:

■ Avoid arching back or performing a pelvic tilt.

■ If you are unable to perform this exercise without the abdomen bulging continue working on the transverse abdominis exercise (page 26) before progressing to this exercise.

BENEFITS:

The rectus abdominis muscle, also known as the 'six pack muscle', engages during this exercise. It also strengthens the iliopsoas, a deep hip muscle.

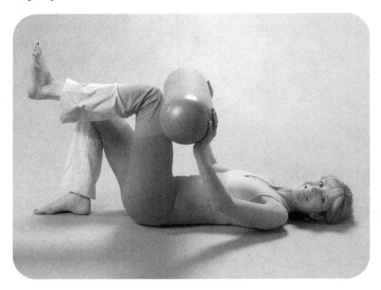

INSTRUCTION:

Lie on back with knees bent. Gently draw lower abdomen toward spine as left knee, hip and ankle are bent to 90 degrees. Place roller on bent knee and hands on either end of roller. Press hands and knee into roller without movement. Hold. Relax and once again press into roller. Repeat with right side.

Ch5 Strengthening

Core Strength Training © *2006 Caroline Corning Creager 1-800-530-6878*

Lower Abdominal Crunch ★★★☆☆

BENEFITS:

This exercise strengthens the rectus abdominis muscle, also known as the 'six pack muscle'.

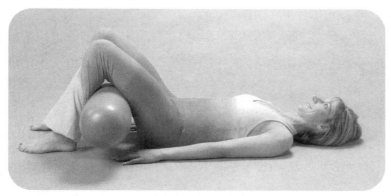

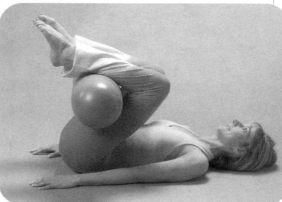

INSTRUCTION:

Lie on back with knees bent and roller positioned between heels and back of thighs. Straighten arms and place next to body and focus eyes on ceiling. Gently draw lower abdomen toward spine and raise knees to chest—squeezing roller between heels and thighs. Maintaining a neutral spine (a position where back is not arched or flat, it is somewhere in between), slowly lower feet to floor.

ROLLERS...

✓ FOAM
✓ INFLATABLE

TARGET AREAS:

Abdominal muscles.

hold:
3 seconds

repeat:
1–3 set(s), 6–10 reps

frequency:
2–3 times per week

HELPFUL HINTS:

- Avoid tipping or tucking chin
- If you are unable to perform this exercise without the abdomen bulging continue working on the *Transverse Abdominis* exercise (page 26) before progressing to this exercise.

93

29

★★★☆☆

Abdominal Crunch

ROLLERS...

X	FOAM
✓	INFLATABLE

It is uncomfortable to use a foam roller.

TARGET AREAS:
Abdominal and neck muscles.

hold:
2 seconds

repeat:
1–2 set(s), 6–10 reps

frequency:
2–3 times per week

notes

BENEFITS:

This exercise strengthens the neck and rectus abdominis muscle, also known as the 'six pack muscle'. It is more difficult to perform than a standard abdominal crunch.

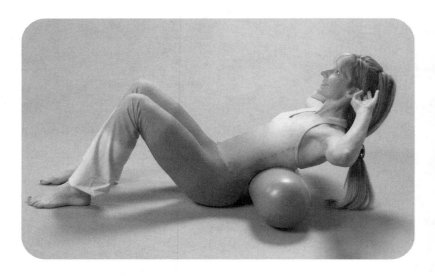

INSTRUCTION: step one

Lie on back with knees bent and roller positioned between hips and lower rib cage. Place unclasped hands behind the head and gently draw lower abdomen toward spine.

Core Strength Training © *2006 Caroline Corning Creager 1-800-530-6878*

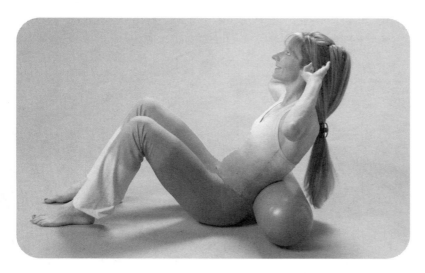

INSTRUCTION:
step two

Slowly raise head toward ceiling focusing eyes on ceiling. Return to starting position.

Avoid tucking or tipping chin

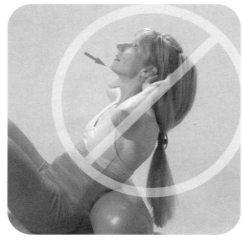

95

exercise

30

★★★☆☆

Oblique Crunch

ROLLERS...

x	FOAM
✓	INFLATABLE

It is uncomfortable to use a foam roller.

TARGET AREAS:

Abdominal and neck muscles.

hold:
2 seconds

repeat:
1–3 set(s), 6–10 reps

frequency:
2–3 times per week

notes

BENEFITS:

This exercise strengthens the neck and oblique abdominal muscles located at the side of the trunk. It tones the muscles underneath the 'love handle' area.

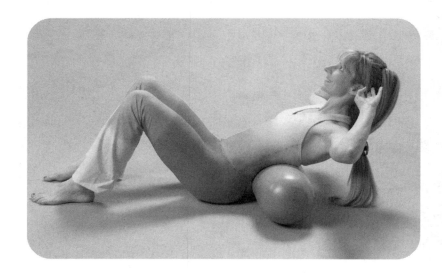

INSTRUCTION: step one

Lie on back with knees bent and roller positioned between hips and lower rib cage. Place unclasped hands behind the head and gently draw lower abdomen toward spine.

96

Ch5 Strengthening

Core Strength Training © *2006 Caroline Corning Creager 1-800-530-6878*

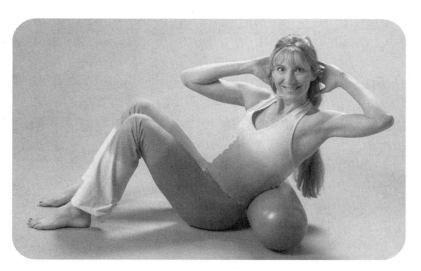

HELPFUL HINTS:

- Avoid tucking or tipping chin back as depicted below

- If you are unable to perform this exercise without the bulging then continue working on the transverse abdominis exercise (page 26) before progressing to this exercise.

INSTRUCTION:
step two

Slowly raise head toward ceiling focusing eyes on ceiling. Return to starting position.

Avoid tucking or tipping chin

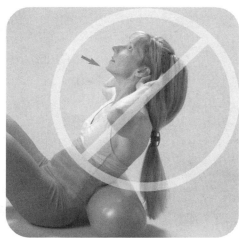

Ch5 Strengthening

31

★★★☆☆

exercise

Sideways Crunch

ROLLERS...

✗	FOAM	
✓	INFLATABLE	

It is uncomfortable to use a foam roller.

TARGET AREAS:

Oblique, neck and abdominal muscles.

hold:
2 seconds

repeat:
1–3 set(s), 6–10 reps

frequency:
2–3 times per week

notes

_____

_____

_____

_____

_____

_____

_____

BENEFITS:

This exercise strengthens the neck and oblique abdominal muscles located at the side of the trunk. It helps tone the muscles underneath the 'love handle' area, and provides a gentle stretch to the low back.

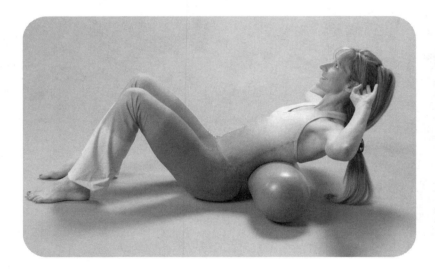

INSTRUCTION: step one

Lie on back with knees bent and roller positioned between hips and lower rib cage. Place unclasped hands behind the head and gently draw lower abdomen toward spine.

98

Ch5 Strengthening

Core Strength Training © 2006 Caroline Corning Creager 1-800-530-6878

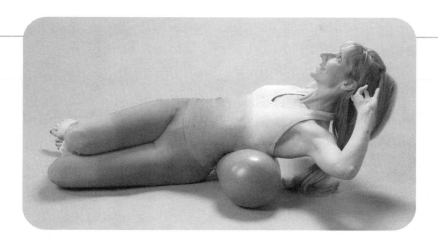

HELPFUL HINTS:

■ Avoid tucking or tipping chin

■ If you are unable to perform this exercise without the bulging then continue working on the transverse abdominis exercise (page 26) before progressing to this exercise.

INSTRUCTION: step two

Slowly rotate knees to the left and lower to the floor.

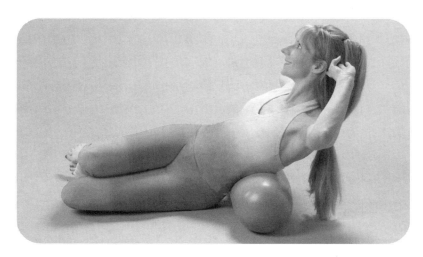

INSTRUCTION: step three

Raise head toward ceiling focusing eyes on ceiling. Slowly return to starting position. Repeat exercise, rotating knees to the right.

Ch5 Strengthening

32

★★☆☆☆

Tummy Trimmin' Trunk Curl–Beginner

ROLLERS...

X	FOAM
✓	INFLATABLE

It is uncomfortable to lie on a foam roller.

TARGET AREAS:

Side abdominal muscles.

hold:
3 seconds

repeat:
1–3 set(s), 5–12 reps each side

frequency:
2–3 times per week

HELPFUL HINTS:

■ Keep a straight line between ankle, hips, shoulders and ears.

■ Neutral spine: A position where back is not arched or flat, it is somewhere in between.

BENEFITS:

The transverse abdominis and oblique muscles must work together in this exercise to keep the abdomen flat. If your abdomen bulges during this exercise, continue working on the Transverse Abdominis exercise on page 26.

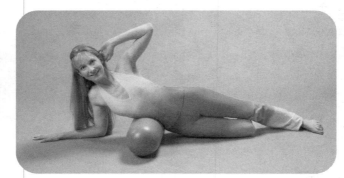

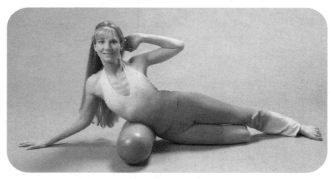

INSTRUCTION:

Lie on side and position roller between lower rib cage and hip. Straighten top leg and bend lower leg. Place right forearm on floor, shoulder aligned with elbow, and left hand behind head. Maintain a neutral spine by gently drawing lower abdomen toward spine. Side bend body by engaging trunk muscles and gently pressing up with right hand. Hold. Return to starting position. Repeat with opposite side.

Ch5 Strengthening

Tummy Trimmin' Trunk Curl–Advanced ★★★★☆

BENEFITS:

The transverse abdominis and oblique muscles must work together in this exercise to keep the abdomen flat. If your abdomen bulges during this exercise, perform the Tummy Trimmin'- Beginner exercise on page 100.

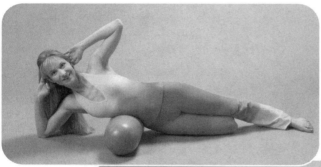

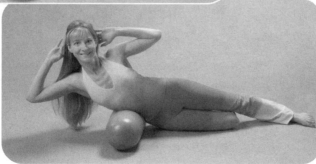

INSTRUCTION:

Lie on side and position roller between lower rib cage and hip. Straighten top leg and bend lower leg. Place unclasped hands behind head. Maintain a neutral spine by gently drawing lower abdomen toward spine. Side bend body after engaging trunk muscles. Hold. Return to starting position. Repeat with opposite side.

ROLLERS...

X	FOAM
✓	INFLATABLE

It is uncomfortable to lie on a foam roller.

TARGET AREAS:
Side abdominal muscles.

hold:
3 seconds

repeat:
1–3 set(s), 5–12 reps each side

frequency:
2–3 times per week

HELPFUL HINTS:

- Keep a straight line between ankle, hips, shoulders and ears.
- Neutral spine: A position where back is not arched or flat, it is somewhere in between.

101

Ch5 Strengthening

Tummy Trimmin' Trunk Curl with

ROLLERS...

| **✗** | FOAM |
| **✓** | INFLATABLE |

It is uncomfortable to lie on a foam roller.

TARGET AREAS:

Side abdominal, outer thigh and hip muscles.

hold:
3 seconds

repeat:
1–3 set(s), 8–12 reps each side

frequency:
2–3 times per week

notes

BENEFITS:

Right-handed people tend to push out their left hip—for women this is often a carry over from holding kids on their hips—which causes the hip muscles to weaken. This exercise will strengthen the outer thigh, hip, and side abdominal muscles.

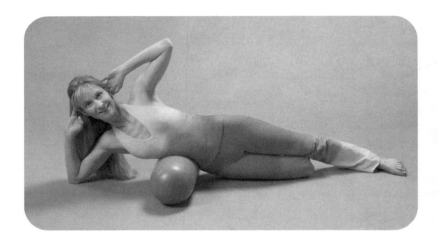

INSTRUCTION: step one

Lie on side and position roller between lower rib cage and hip. Straighten top leg and bend lower leg. Maintain a neutral spine by gently drawing lower abdomen toward spine.

Leg Raise

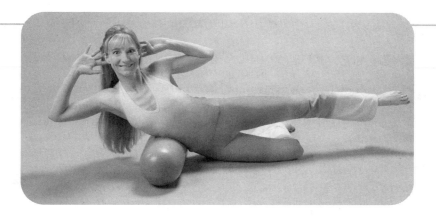

INSTRUCTION: step two

Raise top leg, with foot parallel to floor, to hip height. Side bend. Hold. Return to starting position. Repeat with opposite leg.

VARIATION:

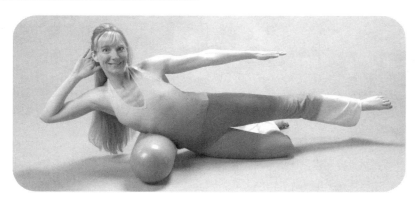

INSTRUCTION:

Follow directions as above however after side bending, straighten top arm over raised leg.

103

Ch5 Strengthening

35

★★★★☆

Abdominal Blaster

TARGET AREAS:

Abdomen, arms, shoulders, back and wrists.

hold:
2 seconds

repeat:
1–3 set(s), 6–10 reps

frequency:
2–3 times per week

notes

BENEFITS:

The body must work as a unit with the exercise, strengthening the arms, shoulders, back, and abdomen in unison. It also provides a gentle low back stretch.

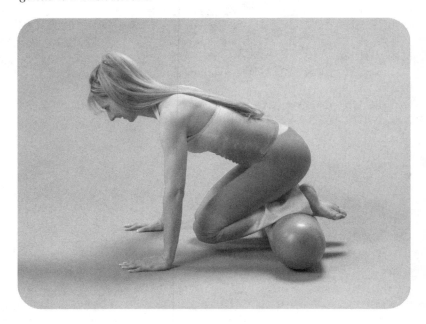

INSTRUCTION: step one

Kneel and position roller under lower legs. Lean forward so hands touch floor with palms flat and fingers pointing forward—wrists should be in alignment with shoulders.

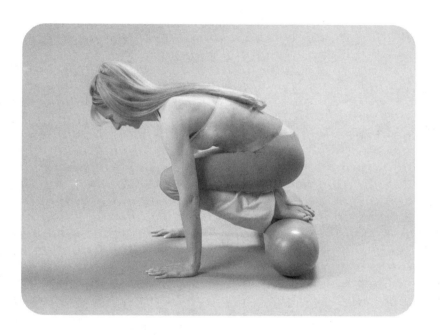

■ Exhale as you draw your knees to chest.

■ If you are unable to perform this exercise without the abdomen sagging then continue working on the *Transverse Abdominis* exercise (page 26) before progressing to this exercise.

■ If you have limited knee range of motion, try performing the *Prone Plank* exercises instead, pages 113-117.

INSTRUCTION: step two

Gently draw lower abdomen toward spine. Rapidly draw knees toward chest as far as possible and return to starting position.

36
★★★★★

Abdominal 'V'

ROLLERS...

✓ FOAM

✓ INFLATABLE

It may be more comfortable to sit on an inflatable roller.

TARGET AREAS:

Abdominal muscles.

hold:
1–3 seconds

repeat:
1–3 set(s), 3–8 reps

frequency:
2–3 times per week

notes

BENEFITS:

Although this exercise requires phenomenal abdominal strength, the goal of this exercise is to work all of your muscles in unison; abdominal, back, neck, arms, and leg muscles. This exercise also improves balance and coordination.

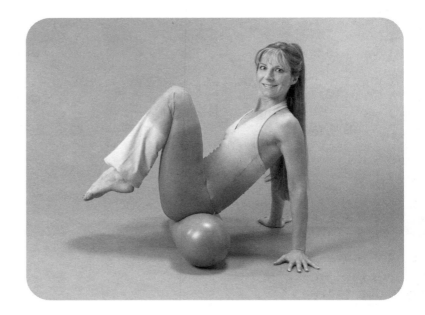

INSTRUCTION: step one

Sit on roller with knees bent and hip-width apart. Maintain a neutral spine by drawing lower abdomen toward spine. Lean body back drawing knees to chest and pointing toes. Place hands, shoulder-width apart, on floor and rotate fingers so they face away from body.

Ch5 Strengthening

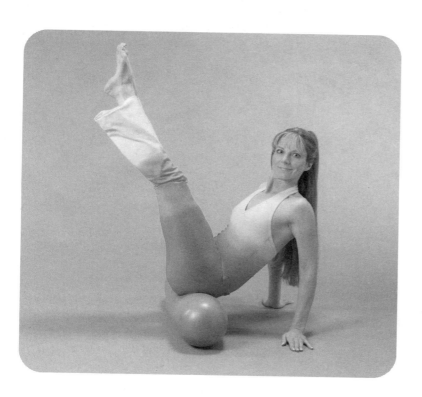

INSTRUCTION: step two

Straighten legs and squeeze shoulder blades together. Keep chest
raised as if suspended from ceiling. Hold. Bend knees and return
to starting position.

Ch5 Strengthening

37
★★★☆☆

Prone Walkout

ROLLERS...

✓ FOAM

✓ INFLATABLE

TARGET AREAS:

Abdomen, arms, wrists, shoulders, neck & chest.

hold:
5–15 seconds

repeat:
1–3 set(s), 3–8 reps

frequency:
3–4 times per week

HELPFUL HINTS:

■ Prevent shoulder blade from winging.

■ Avoid tucking or tipping chin back.

■ Neutral spine: A position where back is not arched or flat, it is somewhere in between.

BENEFITS:

This exercise strengthens the upper body and neck. It also requires good shoulder blade coordination.

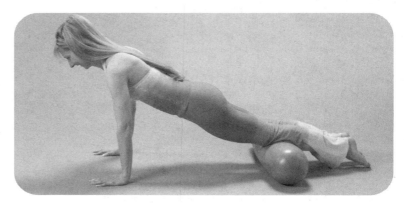

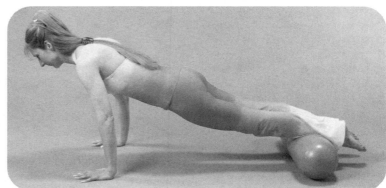

INSTRUCTION:

Kneel and position roller under lower legs. Lean forward so hands touch floor with palms flat and fingers pointing forward. Gently draw lower abdomen toward spine and straighten legs. Walk hands out away from roller until feet are on top of roller.

Ch5 Strengthening

Prone Tuck

★★★☆☆

BENEFITS:

This exercise strengthens the upper body, neck and hips. It also requires good shoulder blade coordination.

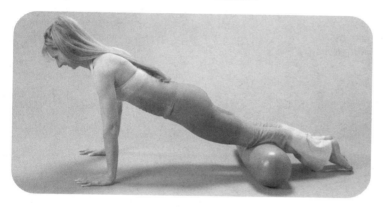

INSTRUCTION:

Kneel and position roller under lower legs. Lean forward so hands touch floor with palms flat and fingers pointing forward—wrists should be in alignment with shoulders. Gently draw lower abdomen toward spine and straighten legs. Draw knees toward chest as far as possible. Return to starting position.

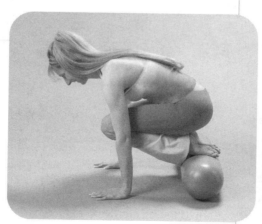

ROLLERS...

✓ FOAM

✓ INFLATABLE

TARGET AREAS:

Abdomen, arms, wrists, shoulders, chest & hips.

hold:
1 second

repeat:
1–3 set(s), 6–12 reps

frequency:
2–3 times per week

HELPFUL HINTS:

- Exhale as you draw your knees to chest.

- If you are unable to perform this exercise without the abdomen sagging continue working on the *Transverse Abdominis* exercise (page 26) before progressing to this exercise.

Ch5 Strengthening

Prone Tuck to Swan Dive

ROLLERS...

✓ FOAM

✓ INFLATABLE

TARGET AREAS:

Abdomen, back buttocks, arms, shoulders, and wrists.

hold:
3 seconds

repeat:
1–3 set(s), 3–8 reps

frequency:
2–3 times per week

notes

_____

_____

_____

_____

BENEFITS:

This is a great dynamic exercise that strengthens both the front and backside of the body. To perform this exercise, the muscles must work together.

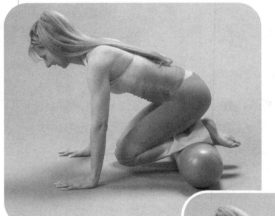

INSTRUCTION:
step one

Kneel and position roller under lower legs. Lean forward so hands touch floor with palms flat and fingers pointing forward—wrists should be in alignment with shoulders. Gently draw lower abdomen toward spine and draw knees toward chest as far as possible.

Ch5 Strengthening

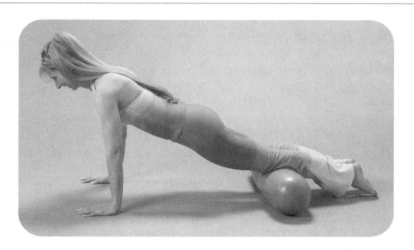

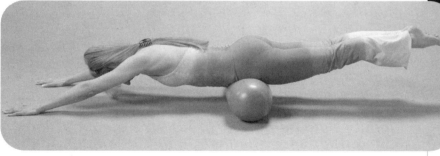

INSTRUCTION: step two

Press feet back and straighten legs. Push body backward with arms, raising feet off floor and lowering head between shoulders. Return to starting position.

Sideways Tuck

TARGET AREAS:

Abdomen, arms, shoulders, and wrists.

hold:
3 seconds

repeat:
1–3 set(s), 6–10 reps

frequency:
2–3 times per week

HELPFUL HINTS:

■ Exhale as you draw your knees to chest.

■ If you are unable to perform this exercise without the abdomen sagging, continue working on the *Transverse Abdominis* exercise (page 26) before progressing to this exercise.

BENEFITS:

This exercise strengthens the back and oblique muscles. The gentle rotation of the back improves back flexibility.

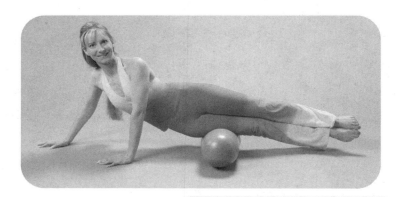

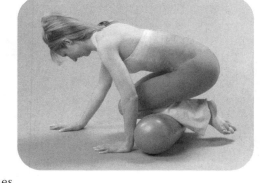

INSTRUCTION:

Kneel and position roller below knees. Straighten arms and place right hand approximately 6 inches in front of left, shoulder width apart, so hands touch floor with palms flat and fingers pointing forward. Gently draw lower abdomen toward spine. Straighten legs by pressing knees back. Rotate hips so only right hip touches roller, keeping legs together. Draw knees toward chest rotating hips so both hips touch roller and return to starting position. Repeat on the opposite side.

Prone Plank–Beginner

★★★☆☆

BENEFITS:

This beginner plank exercise is great for preparing the body for the more advanced prone exercises and improving core muscle strength. It also strengthens the abdominal and neck muscles against gravity. If you are unable to draw the lower abdomen toward the spine in this position, continue working on the Transverse Abdominis exercise on page 26.

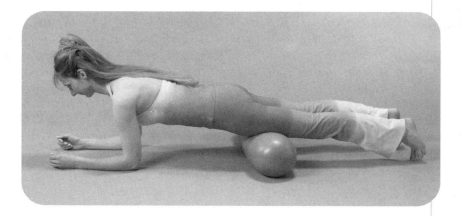

INSTRUCTION:

Lie on abdomen with roller positioned beneath upper thighs. Bend elbows and place forearms on floor. Gently draw lower abdomen toward spine and raise pelvis off floor. Hold. Return to the starting position.

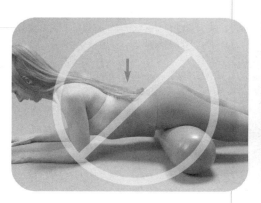

ROLLERS...

✓ FOAM

✓ INFLATABLE

TARGET AREAS:

Abdomen, back, buttocks, neck and shoulders.

hold:
3–15 seconds

repeat:
1–3 set(s), 3–8 reps

frequency:
3–4 times per week

HELPFUL HINTS:

- Avoid rounding back and neck.
- Avoid arching backward and tipping chin back as depicted.
- Neutral spine: A position where back is not arched or flat, it is somewhere in between.

Ch5 Strengthening

Prone Plank–Advanced

ROLLERS...

✓ FOAM
✓ INFLATABLE

TARGET AREAS:

Abdomen, back, inner thighs, neck and shoulders.

hold:
3–15 seconds

repeat:
1–3 set(s), 3–8 reps

frequency:
2–3 times per week

HELPFUL HINTS:

■ Avoid arching back.
■ Avoid tucking or tipping chin back.
■ Maintain a neutral neck and spine.

BENEFITS:

This is a great exercise to strengthen the core, shoulder girdle and inner thighs. In the prone plank position it is usually easier to ascertain whether or not the transverse abdominis requires additional work—the abdomen will "hang out" if it is weak.

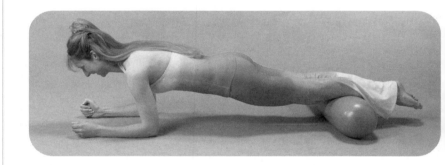

INSTRUCTION:

Lie on abdomen with roller positioned beneath shins. Bend elbows and place forearms on floor. Gently draw lower abdomen toward spine and raise pelvis off floor. Hold. Return to the starting position.

Ch5 Strengthening

Core Strength Training © 2006 Caroline Corning Creager 1-800-530-6878

Prone Plank with Leg Raise

BENEFITS:

This difficult exercise strengthens the core, shoulder girdle and back of thighs. The Prone Plank with Leg Raise works the front and back of body at the same time—okay, it works just about ALL the muscle groups in the body!

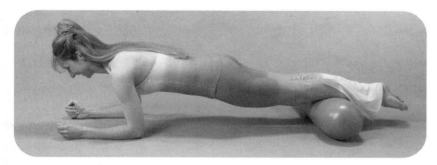

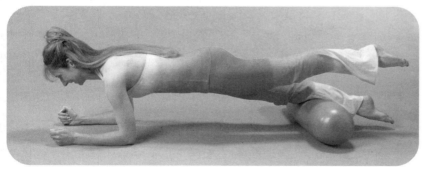

INSTRUCTION:

Lie on abdomen with roller positioned beneath lower legs. Bend elbows and place forearms on floor. Gently draw lower abdomen toward spine and raise pelvis off floor. Raise left foot several inches off roller. Maintain a neutral neck and spine position. Hold. Return to starting position and repeat with opposite leg.

ROLLERS...

✓ FOAM

✓ INFLATABLE

TARGET AREAS:

Neck and Back.

hold:
3–5 seconds

repeat:
1–3 set(s), 3–8 reps each side

frequency:
2–3 times per week

HELPFUL HINTS:

■ Avoid tucking or tipping chin back.

■ Maintain good hip alignment by not allowing heel to rotate in or out.

115

44

★★★★★

Prone Plank with Elbows on Roller

ROLLERS...

x	FOAM
✓	INFLATABLE

It is uncomfortable to place forearms on a foam roller.

TARGET AREAS:

Abdomen, back, inner thighs, and shoulders.

hold:
3–10 seconds

repeat:
1–3 set(s), 3–8 reps

frequency:
2–3 times per week

HELPFUL HINTS:

- Avoid arching back.
- Avoid tucking or tipping chin back.
- Maintain a neutral neck and spine.

BENEFITS:

This exercise improves balance and strengthens the core, shoulder girdle, and inner thighs. It is more difficult than the Prone Plank with Leg Raise exercise, because it is more difficult to stabilize the trunk and shoulders when the forearms are on the inflatable roller.

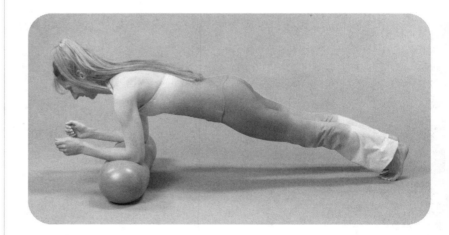

INSTRUCTION:

Kneel. Lean forward and place forearms on roller, maintaining elbow alignment below shoulders. Gently draw lower abdomen toward spine and straighten legs. Maintain a neutral neck and spine position. Hold. Return to starting position.

45

Prone Plank with Elbows on Roller & Leg Raise ★★★★★

BENEFITS:

This exercise improves balance and strengthens the core, shoulder girdle, buttock and back of thighs. It is more difficult than the Prone Plank with Leg Raise exercise, because it is more difficult to stabilize the trunk and shoulders when forearms are on the inflatable roller.

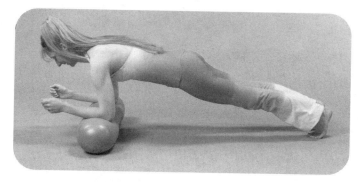

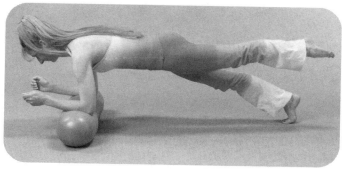

INSTRUCTION:

Follow directions at left, and raise left foot to hip height. Maintain a neutral neck and spine position. Hold. Return to starting position and repeat with opposite leg.

ROLLERS...

X	FOAM
✓	INFLATABLE

It is uncomfortable to place forearms on a foam roller.

TARGET AREAS:

Abdomen, back, inner thighs, and shoulders.

hold:
3 seconds

repeat:
1–2 set(s), 3–8 reps each side

frequency:
daily

HELPFUL HINTS:

- Avoid arching back.
- Avoid tucking or tipping chin back.
- Maintain good hip alignment by not allowing heel to rotate in or out.

Ch5 Strengthening

46
★★★★★

Trunk Scissor Twist

ROLLERS...

✓ FOAM

✓ INFLATABLE

TARGET AREAS:

Abdomen, back, buttocks, neck and shoulders.

hold:
3 seconds

repeat:
1–3 set(s), 3–5 reps each side

frequency:
2–3 times per week

notes

BENEFITS:

This difficult exercise strengthens the core, shoulder girdle, and back of thighs. It gently rotates the spine and works the front and backside of the body at the same time—okay, it's another exercise that works just about ALL the muscle groups in the body!

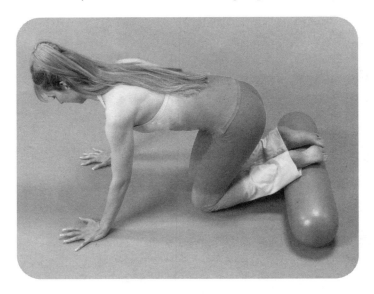

INSTRUCTION: step one

Kneel and position roller beneath feet. Lean forward and place hands on floor. Gently draw lower abdomen toward spine.

Ch5 Strengthening

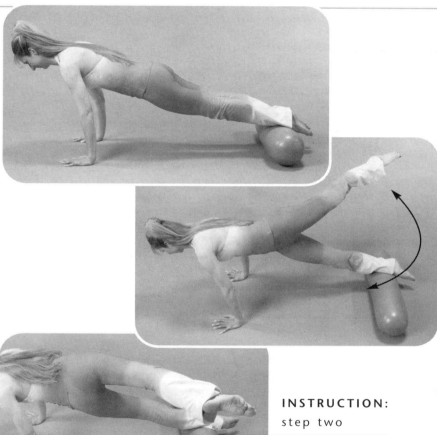

INSTRUCTION: step two

Straighten legs and assume a push-up position.

INSTRUCTION: step three

Slowly raise the left leg and scissor it across opposite leg—rotation occurring at the hip from a horizontal position to a more vertical position. Hold. Return to starting position and repeat with opposite leg.

Ch5 Strengthening

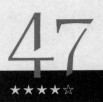
Trunk Twist

TARGET AREAS:

Abdominal, arms, back, & shoulder muscles.

hold:
3 seconds

repeat:
1–3 set(s), 3–8 reps

frequency:
2–3 times per week

notes

_____

_____

_____

_____

BENEFITS:

The Trunk Twist provides a gentle stretch to the low back while working the oblique and transverse abdominis muscles.

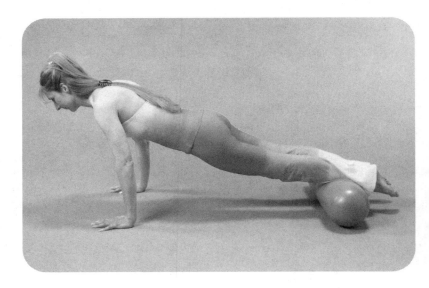

INSTRUCTION: step one

Kneel and position roller beneath ankles. Lean forward so arms are beneath shoulders and hands are shoulder-width apart. Gently draw lower abdomen toward spine and maintain a neutral spine. Straighten legs and assume a push-up position.

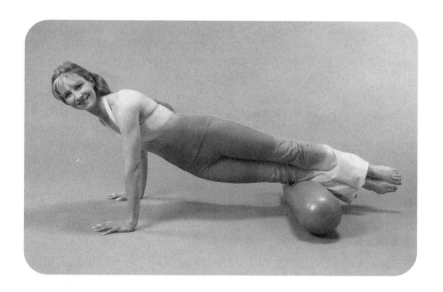

HELPFUL HINTS:

■ Avoid hyper-extending elbows by keeping a slight bend in them.

■ Avoid arching or rounding back.

■ Avoid tucking or tipping chin back.

■ Neutral spine: A position where back is not arched or flat, it is somewhere in between.

INSTRUCTION: step two

Gently rotate hips, head and trunk to the left 90 degrees. Return to a push-up position. Repeat with opposite side.

Supine Plank

ROLLERS...

✓ FOAM

✓ INFLATABLE

TARGET AREAS:

Abdomen, back, buttocks, and shoulders.

hold:
3 seconds

repeat:
1–3 sets, 3–8 reps

frequency:
2–3 times per week

notes

BENEFITS:

The Supine Plank strengthens the core muscles and increases chest and shoulder flexibility. If you have tight chest and shoulder muscles, this exercise will be difficult to perform in good alignment.

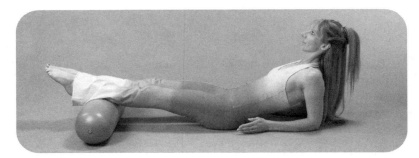

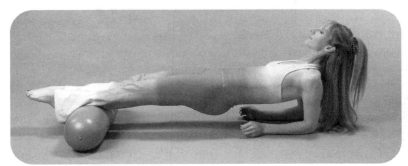

INSTRUCTION:

Sit on floor and place roller horizontally under heels. Recline back with bent elbows, aligning elbows underneath shoulders and focusing eyes on ceiling. Gently draw lower abdomen toward spine and raise buttocks off floor. Hold. Return to starting position.

Supine Plank with Leg Raise ★★★★☆

BENEFITS:

The Supine Plank improves balance, strengthens the core muscles, and increases chest and shoulder flexibility. If you have tight chest and shoulder muscles, this exercise will be difficult to perform in good alignment.

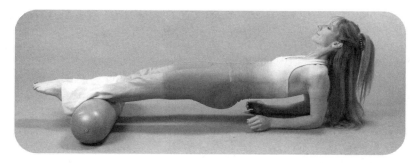

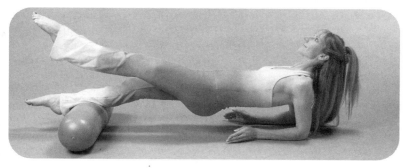

INSTRUCTION:

Sit on floor and place roller horizontally under heels. Recline back with bent elbows, aligning elbows underneath shoulders and focusing eyes on ceiling. Gently draw lower abdomen toward spine and raise buttocks off floor. Raise left straight leg off roller. Hold. Return to starting position. Repeat with opposite leg.

ROLLERS...

✓ FOAM
✓ INFLATABLE

TARGET AREAS:

Abdomen, back, buttocks, and shoulders.

hold:
3–5 seconds

repeat:
1–3 set(s), 3–8 reps each side

frequency:
2–3 times per week

HELPFUL HINTS:

- Avoid rounding back and neck.
- Avoid tucking or tipping chin back.
- Neutral spine: A position where back is not arched or flat, it is somewhere in between.

Ch5 Strengthening

50

★★★★☆

Advanced Supine Plank

BENEFITS:

This exercise improves core strength and flexibility in the chest and shoulders. Men tend to have strong chest muscles making them less flexible in this area. Hence, men may find this exercise difficult to perform in good form.

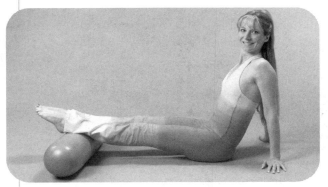

INSTRUCTION:
step one

Sit on floor with legs straight and roller positioned horizontally under heels. Straighten arms. Place hands behind back on floor with fingers rotated out away from body. Maintain a neutral spine by drawing lower abdomen toward spine.

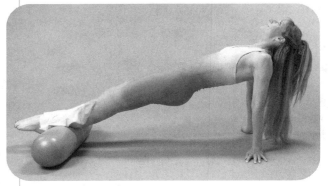

INSTRUCTION: step two

Raise buttocks off floor and maintain a line between shoulders hips, and ankles. Keep hands aligned underneath shoulders and eyes focused on ceiling. Hold. Return to starting position.

Advanced Supine Plank with Leg Raise ★★★★★

BENEFITS:

The supine plank with leg raise improves balance, strengthens the core muscles, and increases chest and shoulder flexibility. If you have tight chest and shoulder muscles, this exercise will be difficult to per-form in good alignment. Try the Chest Stretch on page 34 prior to performing this exercise.

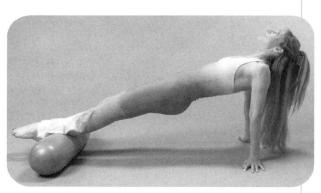

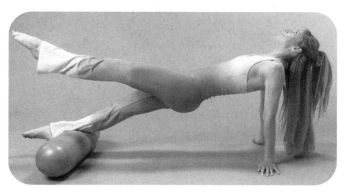

INSTRUCTION:

Follow directions for Advanced Supine Plank. Raise straight left leg off roller. Hold. Return to starting position. Repeat with opposite leg.

ROLLERS...

✓ FOAM

✓ INFLATABLE

TARGET AREAS:

Abdomen, back, buttocks, hips, legs and shoulders.

hold:
3 seconds

repeat:
1–3 set(s), 3–8 reps each side

frequency:
daily

HELPFUL HINTS:

■ Avoid tucking or tipping chin back.

■ Neutral spine: A position where back is not arched or flat, it is somewhere in between.

Ch5 Strengthening

Back Extension–Beginner

ROLLERS...

✗	FOAM
✓	INFLATABLE

It is uncomfortable to lie on a foam roller.

TARGET AREAS:

Lower back, abdomen, and buttock muscles.

hold:
3 seconds

repeat:
1–3 set(s), 6–12 reps

frequency:
2–3 times per week

HELPFUL HINTS:

■ As the exercise becomes easier rely less on pressing up with your hands and more on your abdominal, back and buttock muscles for the motion.

■ Avoid arching back.

BENEFITS:

Pressing up with the hands makes the exercise easier than placing hands behind the back. It also can relieve pressure on the lumbar discs and stretch the front muscles.

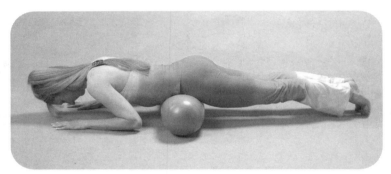

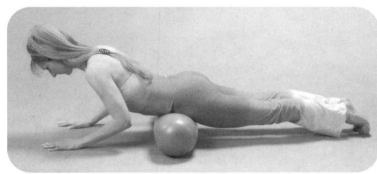

INSTRUCTION:

Lie on abdomen with roller positioned between lower ribs and hips. Place hands on floor in front of roller. Gently draw lower abdomen toward spine and lightly press body up with hands. Maintain a neutral neck and spine position (a position where back and neck are not arched or flat, they are somewhere in between). Hold. Slowly lower body to starting position.

Back Extension–Advanced

★★★★★

BENEFITS:

This exercise improves flexibility and strength in the lower back.

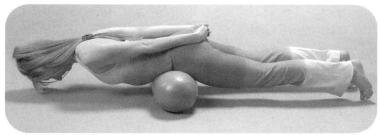

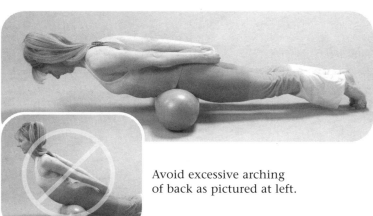

Avoid excessive arching
of back as pictured at left.

ROLLERS...

| x | FOAM |
| ✓ | INFLATABLE |

*It is uncomfortable to
lie on a foam roller.*

TARGET AREAS:

*Lower back,
abdomen, and
buttock muscles.*

hold:
3 seconds

repeat:
1–3 sets, 3–8 reps

frequency:
2–3 times per week

HELPFUL HINTS:

■ Avoid excessive
arching of the
back as depict-
ed at left. This
motion places
too much
strain on the
lower back
and discs.

INSTRUCTION:

Lie on abdomen with roller positioned between lower ribs and
hips. Grasp hands behind back. Gently draw lower abdomen
toward spine and raise body up away from floor. Maintain a
neutral neck and spine position (A position where back and
neck are not arched or flat, they are somewhere in between).
Hold. Slowly lower body to starting position.

127

54

★★★★★

Back Extension with Rotation

ROLLERS...

 X   FOAM

✓   INFLATABLE

It is uncomfortable to lie on a foam roller.

TARGET AREAS:

Lower back, abdomen, and buttock muscles.

hold:
3 seconds

repeat:
1–3 set(s), 3–8 reps

frequency:
2–3 times per week

notes

BENEFITS:

This difficult exercise improves flexibility and strength in the lower back and side trunk muscles.

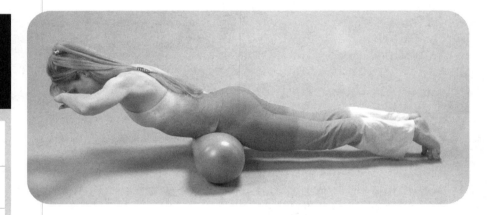

INSTRUCTION: step one

Lie on abdomen with roller positioned between lower ribs and hips. Place back side of left hand on forehead, as if saluting, and right hand by side of body. Gently draw lower abdomen toward spine and raise body up away from floor. Maintain a neutral neck and spine position.

Core Strength Training © 2006 Caroline Corning Creager 1-800-530-6878

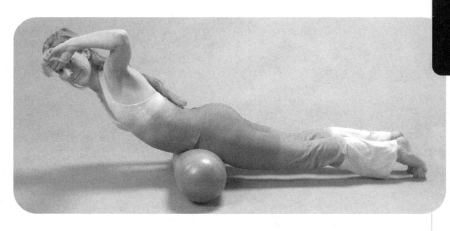

INSTRUCTION: step two

Rotate trunk to the left. Slowly lower body to starting position. Repeat on opposite side.

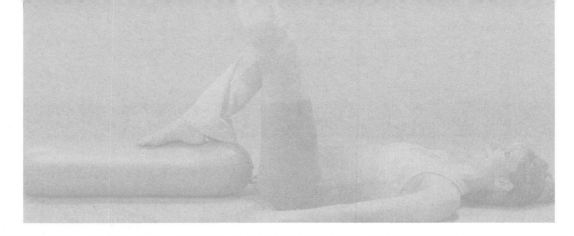

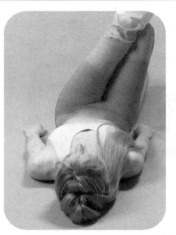

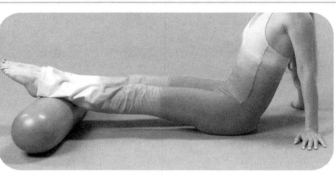

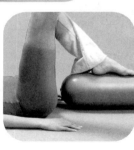

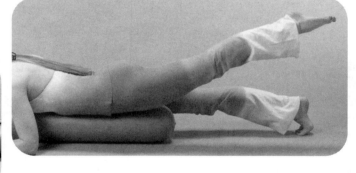

Lower Body Exercises

Lower
Body
Exercises

Straight Leg Hip Lift

ROLLERS...

✓ FOAM

✓ INFLATABLE

TARGET AREAS:

Buttock and back of thigh muscles.

hold:
5 seconds

repeat:
1–3 sets, 6–12 reps

frequency:
2–3 times per week

HELPFUL HINTS:

- If your knees hyperextend, bend backward, perform the *Bent Knee Hip Lift* **initially on page 135.**

- **Avoid arching back. This places increased stress on the lower back and discs.**

BENEFITS:

This leg and buttock strengthening exercise is a great basic exercise — just about anyone can perform it.

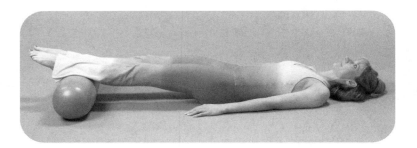

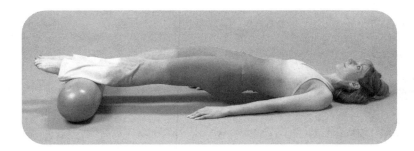

INSTRUCTION:

Lie on back and place feet on roller. Maintain a neutral spine by gently drawing lower abdomen in toward spine (a position where back is not arched or flat, but somewhere in between). Keeping legs straight, lift hips off floor. Return to starting position.

Ch5 Strengthening

Core Strength Training © *2006 Caroline Corning Creager* 1-800-530-6878

Straight Leg Hip Lift with Feet Crossed ★☆☆☆☆

BENEFITS:

This exercise helps improve balance as well as strengthening the buttocks, back, and thighs.

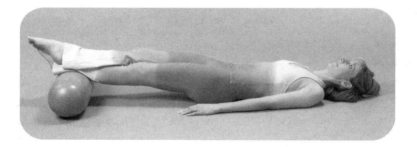

INSTRUCTION:

Follow directions from previous exercise, however cross right foot over the left and lift hips off floor. Return to starting position. After completing one set, cross left foot over right and perform another set.

ROLLERS...

✓ FOAM

✓ INFLATABLE

TARGET AREAS:

Buttock and back of thigh muscles.

hold:
3-8 seconds

repeat:
1–3 sets, 6–12 reps each side

frequency:
2–3 times per week

HELPFUL HINTS:

- If your knees hyperextend, bend backward, perform the *Bent Knee Hip Lift* on page 135.
- Avoid arching back. This places increased stress on the lower back and discs.

133

Ch5 Strengthening

57

★★★☆☆

Straight Leg Hip Lift with Leg Raise

exercise

ROLLERS...

✓ FOAM

✓ INFLATABLE

TARGET AREAS:

Buttock and back of thigh muscles.

hold:
3–5 seconds

repeat:
1-3 sets, 3–8 reps each side

frequency:
2–3 times per week

HELPFUL HINTS:

■ If your knees hyperextend, bend backward, perform the *Bent Knee Hip Lift* on page 135.

■ Avoid arching back. This places increased stress on the lower back and discs.

BENEFITS:

This exercise helps stabilize the pelvic muscles, improves balance, and is more difficult than the previous two exercises. This exercise is typically easier on one side indicating you may have a hip strength imbalance. Improve hip strength on the weaker side by increasing the number of repetitions you perform.

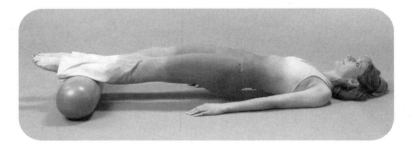

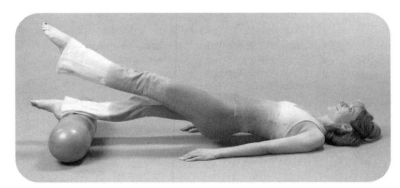

INSTRUCTION:

Follow directions from Straight Leg Hip Lift, page 132. Keeping legs straight, lift hips off floor and raise right leg 6 inches off of roller. Hold: 3 seconds. Return to starting position. Keeping legs straight, lift hips off floor and raise left leg 6 inches off of roller. Return to starting position.

134

Ch5 Strengthening

Bent Knee Hip Lift

★☆☆☆☆

BENEFITS:

This exercise strengthens the hamstring or back of thigh muscles. If your knees tend to hyperextend, or bend backward, it is better to perform this exercise than the Straight Leg Hip Lift on page 132.

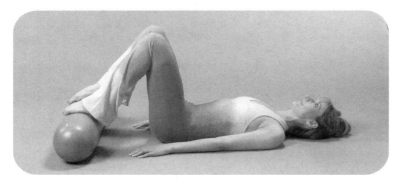

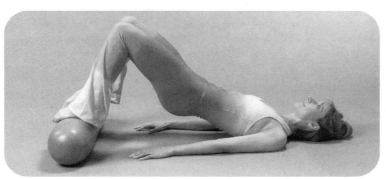

INSTRUCTION:

Lie on back with knees bent and roller positioned under feet. Maintain a neutral spine by drawing lower abdomen towards spine. Lift hips off floor several inches. Lower hips to floor.

ROLLERS...

✓ FOAM

✓ INFLATABLE

TARGET AREAS:
Lower back, buttock, calf, and thigh muscles.

hold:
3 seconds

repeat:
*1–2 set(s),
8–12 reps*

frequency:
2–3 times per week

HELPFUL HINTS:

■ Avoid raising hips too high. This places increased stress on the neck, back and discs.

■ Neutral spine: A position where back is not arched or flat, it is somewhere in between.

Ch5 Strengthening

59

★★☆☆☆

Hamstring Curl

TARGET AREAS:

Lower back, buttock, calf, and thigh muscles.

hold:
3–5 seconds

repeat:
1–3 set(s), 6–12 reps

frequency:
2–3 times per week

HELPFUL HINTS:

■ Avoid arching back. This places increased stress on the lower back and discs.

■ Neutral spine: A position where back is not arched or flat, but somewhere in between.

BENEFITS:

The hamstring muscles located in the back of the thighs are weaker than the quadriceps, the front thigh muscles. This exercise will improve hamstring strength and make walking uphill easier.

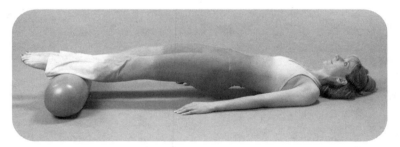

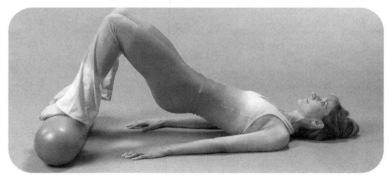

INSTRUCTION:

Lie on back with straight legs. Place heels on roller. Maintain a neutral spine by drawing lower abdomen towards spine. Lift hips off floor. Draw knees toward chest. Straighten legs and lower hips to floor.

One-Legged Hamstring Curl

★★★☆☆

BENEFITS:

Most people have one leg that is stronger than the other. It will become evident with this exercise, because typically you will perform fewer repetitions on that side. Improve strength on the weaker side by increasing the number of repetitions you perform.

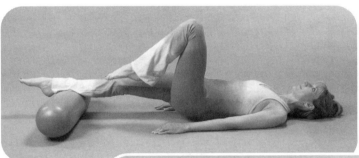

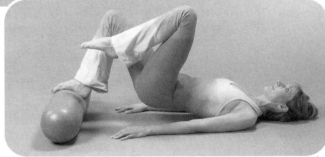

INSTRUCTION:

Lie on back and place right heel on roller. Bend left knee. Maintain a neutral spine by drawing lower abdomen towards spine. Lift hips off floor and draw right knee toward chest. Straighten right leg and lower hips to floor. Repeat with opposite side.

ROLLERS...

✓ FOAM

✓ INFLATABLE

TARGET AREAS:

Lower back, buttock, calf, and thigh muscles.

hold:
3–5 seconds

repeat:
1–3 set(s),
3–8 reps each side

frequency:
2–3 times per week

HELPFUL HINTS:

- Avoid arching back. This places increased stress on the lower back and discs.
- Neutral spine: A position where back is not arched or flat, it is somewhere in between.

Ch5 Strengthening

Hip Lift on Roller

ROLLERS...

✓ FOAM

✓ INFLATABLE

TARGET AREAS:

Back, buttocks, and back of thigh muscles.

hold:
3–5 seconds

repeat:
1–3 set(s), 5–8 reps

frequency:
2–3 times per week

HELPFUL HINTS:

- Avoid raising hips too high to prevent placing too much stress on the neck.

- Neutral spine: A position where back is not arched or flat, it is somewhere in between.

BENEFITS:

Although this exercise is performed while lying on your back, it strengthens the majority of your major muscle groups. It is unique because it also helps stabilize the mid back and scapular muscles.

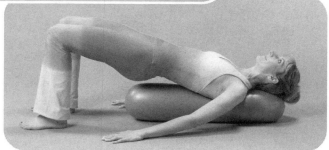

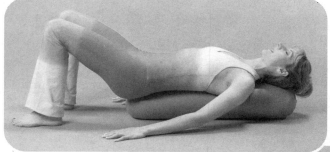

INSTRUCTION:

Lie on side with knees bent. Roll head and back onto roller with feet flat on floor. Focusing eyes on ceiling, gently draw lower abdomen toward spine and raise buttocks off floor. Maintain a neutral spine. Hold. Return to starting position.

138

Knee Raise on Roller

 ★☆☆☆☆

BENEFITS:

Most people have one leg that is stronger than the other. It will become evident with this exercise, because one hip may dip — try to keep them level.

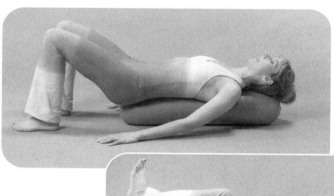

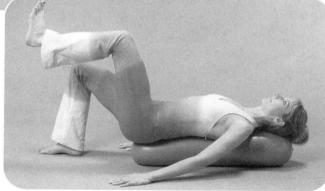

INSTRUCTION:

Lie on side with knees bent. Roll head and back onto roller with feet flat on floor. Focusing eyes on ceiling, gently draw lower abdomen toward spine. Raise left knee and hip to 90 degrees and flex foot. Maintain a neutral spine and keep hips level. Hold. Lower right foot to floor. Repeat with opposite side.

ROLLERS...

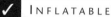

✓ FOAM

✓ INFLATABLE

TARGET AREAS:

Back, buttocks, and back of thigh muscles.

hold:
3–5 seconds

repeat:
1–3 set(s), 3–8 reps on each side

frequency:
2–3 times per week

HELPFUL HINTS:

- Avoid raising hips too high to prevent placing too much stress on the neck.
- Neutral spine: A position where back is not arched or flat, it is somewhere in between.

139

Ch5 Strengthening

Straight Leg Raise

ROLLERS...

✓ FOAM

✓ INFLATABLE

TARGET AREAS:

Front thigh, hip, and abdominal muscles.

hold:
3 seconds

repeat:
1–3 set(s), 6–12 reps each side

frequency:
2–3 times per week

notes

BENEFITS:

This exercise strengthens the quadricep or front thigh muscles. This is also a great exercise for individuals who have weak knees. It requires a lot of strength and coordination to keep your foot from falling off the roller.

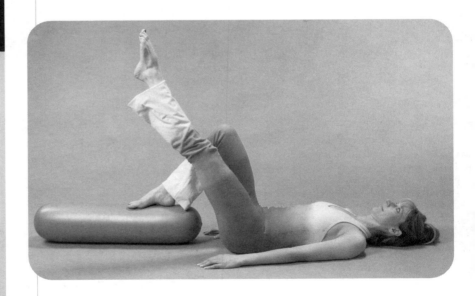

INSTRUCTION: step one

Lie on back with knees bent and roller positioned under right foot as shown. Maintain a neutral spine by drawing lower abdomen towards spine. Straighten left leg and raise, with toes pointed, off floor. Hold.

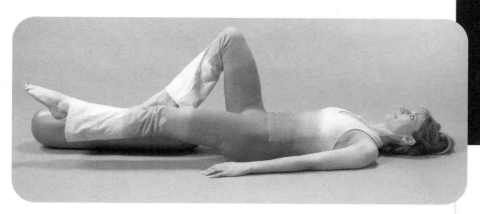

INSTRUCTION: step two

Lower leg, however just before touching floor raise leg up again.
Repeat with right leg.

Ch5 Strengthening

64

Leg Circle

ROLLERS...

✓ FOAM

✓ INFLATABLE

TARGET AREAS:

Front thigh, hip, and abdominal muscles.

hold:
1 second

repeat:
1–3 set(s), 8–12 reps each direction and side

frequency:
2–3 times per week

notes

BENEFITS:

This exercise improves flexibility in the hip joints and strengthens the hip and quadricep (front thigh) muscles. It also requires a lot of abdominal strength to keep your body from moving.

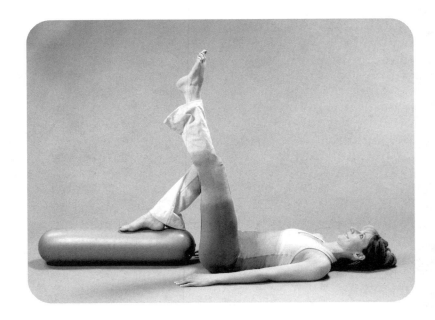

INSTRUCTION: step one

Lie back with knee bent and roller positioned under right foot as shown. Straighten left leg and raise, with toes pointed and turned out off floor.

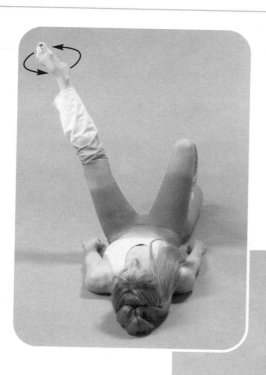

INSTRUCTION:

step two

Make small circles
with left foot. Reverse
directions of circles.
Repeat with right leg.

143

Ch5 Strengthening

65

★★☆☆☆ **Booty Buster Leg Raise**

ROLLERS...

✓ FOAM
✓ INFLATABLE

It may be uncomfortable to lie with abdomen on the foam roller. HOWEVER, using a half foam roller with flat surface up is a comfortable foam roller alternative.

TARGET AREAS:

Buttocks and back of thighs.

hold:
3–5 seconds

repeat:
1–3 set(s), 6–12 reps each side

frequency:
2–3 times per week

notes

BENEFITS:

This exercise strengthens the buttock and hamstring (back of thigh muscles). It also teaches you to move the hip independent of the pelvis and spine, and stretches muscles in the front of the hip.

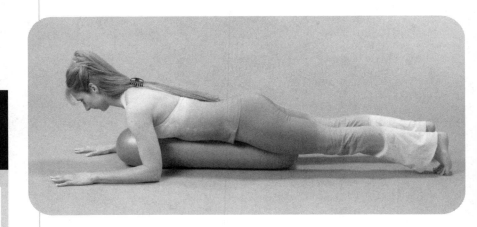

INSTRUCTION: step one

Kneel. Lean forward and place forearms on floor and roller underneath chest and abdomen.

144

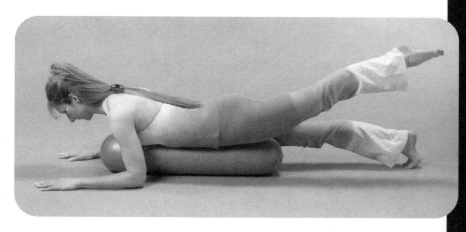

HELPFUL HINTS:

■ Avoid raising leg too high or it will cause the lower back to arch.

■ Maintain good hip alignment by not allowing heel to rotate in or out.

■ Neutral neck and spine: A position where back and neck are not arched or flat, they are somewhere in between.

INSTRUCTION: step two

Gently draw lower abdomen toward spine and raise left leg with toes pointed. Maintain a neutral neck and spine position. Hold. Return to starting position. Repeat with opposite leg.

Ch5 Strengthening

Booty Buster Knee Bend

ROLLERS...

✓ FOAM

✓ INFLATABLE

It may be uncomfortable to lie with abdomen on the foam roller. HOWEVER, using a half foam roller with flat surface up is a comfortable foam roller alternative.

TARGET AREAS:

Buttocks and back of thighs.

hold:
3 seconds

repeat:
1–3 set(s), 6–12 reps each side

frequency:
2–3 times per week

notes

_____

_____

_____

_____

_____

BENEFITS:

The knee-flexed booty buster variation will work the soleus or inner calf muscle. This muscle is often weak in people who experience shin splints.

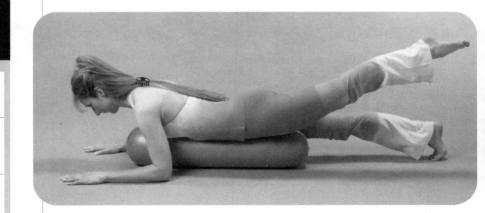

INSTRUCTION:

step one

Kneel. Lean forward and place forearms on floor and roller underneath chest and abdomen. Gently draw lower abdomen toward spine and raise left leg with toes pointed (left) or flexed (right).

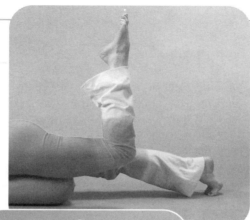

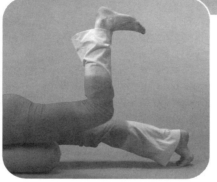

INSTRUCTION:

step two

Bend knee to 90 degrees (above) or as far as you can. Maintain a neutral neck and spine position. Hold. Return to starting position. Repeat with opposite leg.

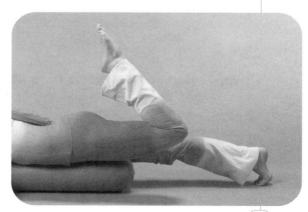

Ch5 Strengthening

67

★☆☆☆☆   Hip Extension

TARGET AREAS:

Buttock, and back of thigh muscles.

hold:
3 seconds

repeat:
1–3 set(s),
6–12 reps

frequency:
2–3 times per week

notes

BENEFITS:

Hip extensions improve strength in the buttock and hamstring (back of thigh) muscles. By flexing toes as depicted in exercise, it lengthens the hamstring muscle causing a greater stretch in the buttock and hamstring area.

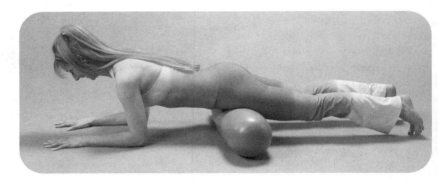

INSTRUCTION: step one

Lie on abdomen with forearms on floor and roller positioned beneath hips. Maintain a neutral neck and spine position by gently drawing lower abdomen toward spine.

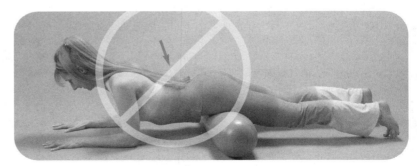

Avoid arching back as pictured above.

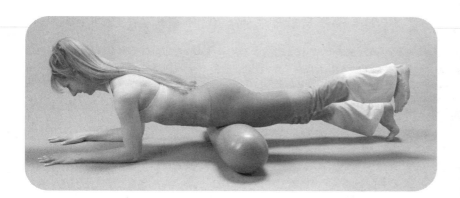

INSTRUCTION: step two

Raise left straight leg, with flexed toes, off floor. Hold. Return to starting position. Repeat with right leg.

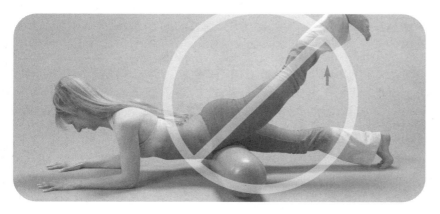

Avoid raising leg too high as pictured above.

Ch5 Strengthening

68

★☆☆☆☆

Heel Pulse

ROLLERS...

✓ FOAM

✓ INFLATABLE

It may be uncomfortable to lie on a foam roller.

TARGET AREAS:

Buttock, inner and outer thigh muscles.

hold:
1 second

repeat:
1–3 set(s), 6–12 reps 3 pulses of heel clicking is one rep

frequency:
2–3 times per week

notes

BENEFITS:

Heel Pulses improve leg coordination and strength in the buttock and thigh muscles.

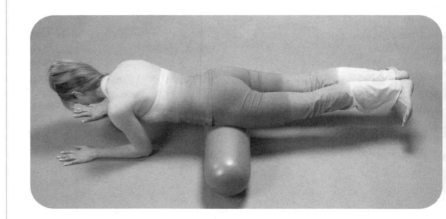

INSTRUCTION: step one

Lie on abdomen with forearms on floor and roller positioned beneath hips. Gently draw lower abdomen toward spine and raise straight legs off floor. Flex toes and rotate feet out so heels touch (the ballet 1st position).

Ch5 Strengthening

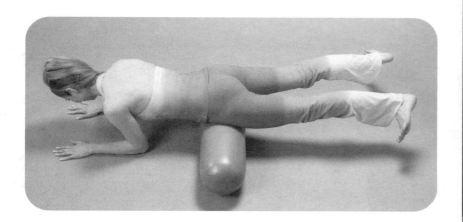

HELPFUL HINTS:

- Avoid rounding or arching back as depicted in photo below.
- Neutral neck and spine: A position where back and neck are not arched or flat, but somewhere in between.

INSTRUCTION: step two

Maintain a neutral neck and spine position. Rapidly open and close legs clicking heels together in pulses of three.

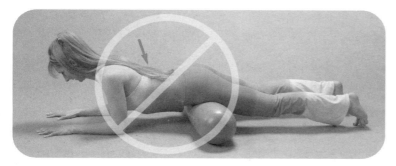

Avoid arching back as pictured above.

Ch5 Strengthening

★☆☆☆☆

Criss Cross Heel Pulse

ROLLERS...

✓ FOAM
✓ INFLATABLE

It may be uncomfortable to lie on a foam roller.

TARGET AREAS:

Buttock, inner and outer thigh muscles.

hold:
1 second

repeat:
1–3 sets,
6–12 reps each side

frequency:
2–3 times per week

notes

_____

_____

_____

_____

_____

BENEFITS:

Criss Cross Heel Pulses improve leg coordination and strength in the buttock and thigh muscles.

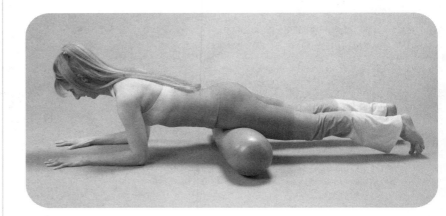

INSTRUCTION: step one

Lie on abdomen with forearms on floor and roller positioned beneath hips. Gently draw lower abdomen toward spine and raise straight legs off floor. Maintain a neutral neck and spine position.

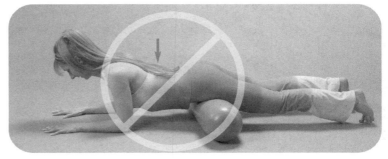

Avoid arching back as pictured above.

INSTRUCTION: step two

Point toes and rapidly cross left foot over right 3 times in a pulsing motion. Switch and rapidly pulse left foot over right 3 times.

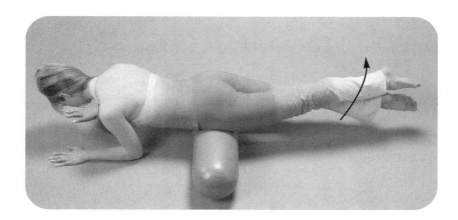

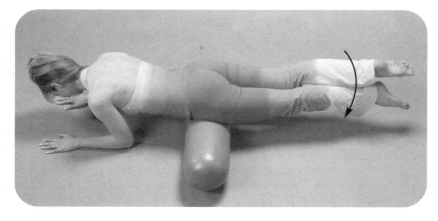

Ch5 Strengthening

★★☆☆☆

Outer Thigh Raise

ROLLERS...

| ✓ | FOAM |
| ✓ | INFLATABLE |

It may be uncomfortable to lie on a foam roller.

TARGET AREAS:

Outer thigh and hip muscles.

hold:
3–5 seconds

repeat:
1–3 set(s), 6–12 reps each side

frequency:
2–3 times per week

HELPFUL HINTS:

■ Keep a straight line between ankle, hips, and shoulders. (Most exercisers tend to bring the ankle in front of hip, this makes the exercise easier but strengthens a different muscle).

BENEFITS:

Right-handed people tend to push out their left hip—for women this is often a carry over from holding kids on their hips—which causes the hip muscles to weaken. This exercise will strengthen the outer thigh and hip muscles.

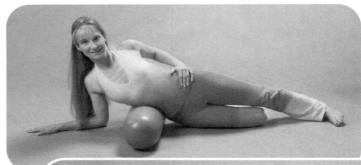

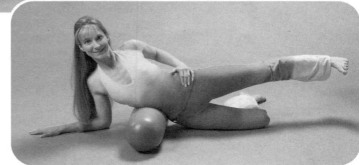

INSTRUCTION:

Lie on side and position roller between lower rib cage and hip. Straighten top leg and bend lower leg. Maintain a neutral spine (a position where back is not arched or flat, it is somewhere in between) by gently drawing lower abdomen toward spine. Raise top leg, with foot parallel to floor, to shoulder height. Hold. Return to starting position. Repeat with opposite leg.

Ch5 Strengthening

Inner Thigh Squeeze

★☆☆☆☆

BENEFITS:

Strengthens and tones inner thigh and pelvic floor muscles. Squeezing the roller may also relieve pain in the pubic bone region by helping to align the pubic bones.

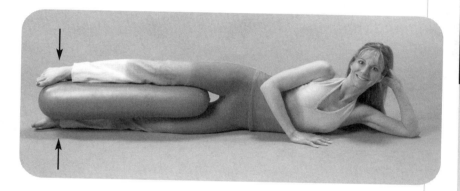

INSTRUCTION:

Lie on side and support head with hand. If supporting your head with your hand is uncomfortable, place your head on a pillow instead. Place roller between inner thighs. Squeeze ankles and inner thighs together. Relax. Repeat.

VARIATION:

Perform exercise as above, however, draw pelvic floor up and in as with a Kegel exercise.

ROLLERS...

✓ FOAM

✓ INFLATABLE

TARGET AREAS:
Inner thigh and pelvic floor muscles.

hold:
3 seconds

repeat:
1–3 set(s), 6–12 reps each side

frequency:
2–3 times per week

HELPFUL HINTS:

■ Keep a straight line between ankle, hips, and shoulders. (Most people tend to bring the ankle in front of hip. This makes the exercise easier but strengthens a different muscle.

exercise

72

★★☆☆☆

Standing Squat

ROLLERS...

✓ FOAM

✓ INFLATABLE

TARGET AREAS:

Buttock and leg muscles.

hold:
3–5 seconds

repeat:
*1–3 set(s),
6–12 reps*

frequency:
2–3 times per week

HELPFUL HINTS:

■ Keep a straight line between ankle, hips, shoulders, and ears in standing position.

■ Neutral neck and spine: A position where back and neck are not arched or flat, they are somewhere in between.

BENEFITS:

Performing a standing squat with a roller in front of your body helps counter balance the weight shift posteriosly (backward). This exercise will strengthen your legs and buttocks.

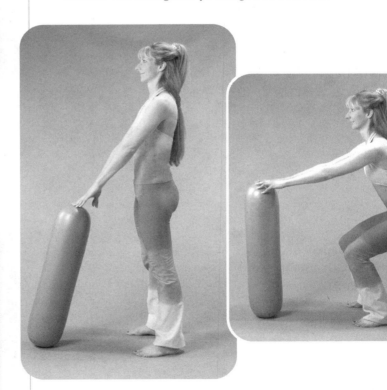

INSTRUCTION:

Stand with roller positioned vertically in front of body and hands on top of roller. Bend knees as roller is gently pressed away from body. Maintain a neutral neck and spine.

Ch5 Strengthening

Standing Plank

★★★★★

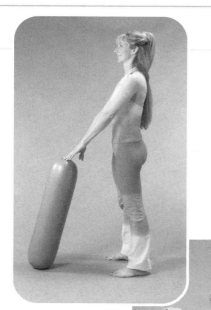

BENEFITS:

This is an advanced exercise that improves core strength balance, and promotes core muscles working synergistically (together)–as they should with any activity you perform thoughout the day.

ROLLERS...

✓ FOAM

✓ INFLATABLE

TARGET AREAS:

Abdomen, back, buttock, and leg muscles.

hold:
3 seconds

repeat:
1–3 set(s), 3–8 reps

frequency:
2–3 times per week

HELPFUL HINTS:

■ In the plank position, keep a straight line between ankle, hips, shoulders, ears and hands.

■ Neutral neck and spine: A position where back and neck are not arched or flat, they are somewhere in between.

INSTRUCTION:

Stand with roller positioned vertically in front of body and hands on top of roller. Gently draw lower abdomen toward spine. Lean forward at waist and press roller away from body. Bend right knee and raise a straight left leg to hip height. Keep foot flexed and toes pointing toward floor. Maintain a neutral neck and spine. Hold. Return to standing position. Perform exercise on opposite leg.

Ch5 Strengthening

74

★★★☆☆

Standing Position on Foam Roller

TARGET AREAS:
Spine, core muscles, and postural muscles.

hold:
1 minute

repeat:
3 reps

frequency:
daily

HELPFUL HINTS:

■ Keep a straight line between ankle, hips, shoulders, and ears.

■ Neutral neck and spine: A position where back and neck are not arched or flat, they are somewhere in between.

BENEFITS:

This exercise strengthens muscles in an optimal position to avoid injury and improves balance reactions.

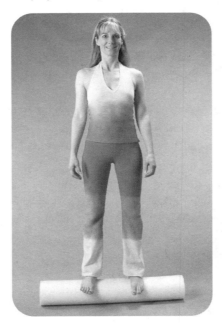
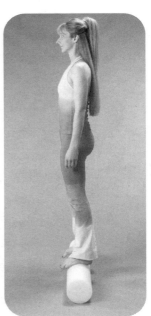

INSTRUCTION:

Stand on roller with feet hip-width apart. Maintain a neutral neck and spine. To keep balance, move arms out away from body.

VARIATION:

A variety of foam roller sizes are available, see page 10. Standing on a half roller is typically easier than standing on a full roller as depicted.

Standing Shoulder to Overhead Lift with Roller ★★★★★

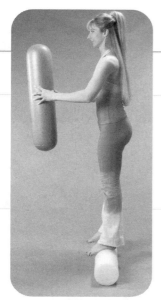

BENEFITS:

Standing on the roller and raising a roller overhead will improve balance and proprioceptive reactions by changing your center of gravity.

INSTRUCTION:

Stand on roller with feet hip-width apart. Grasp second roller and hold it in front of body. Raise arms overhead. Maintain a neutral neck and spine (a position where back and neck are not arched or flat, they are somewhere in between). Lower arms and return to starting position.

Avoid arching back as pictured below.

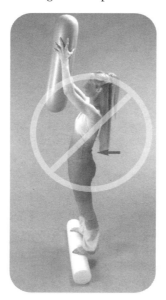

ROLLERS...

✓	FOAM
✗	INFLATABLE

Standing on an inflatable roller is not safe.

TARGET AREAS:

Arms, back, and leg muscles.

hold:
3 seconds

repeat:
1–3 set(s), 3–8 reps

frequency:
2–3 times per week

HELPFUL HINTS:

■ Avoid arching back as you raise your arms overhead as in photo at left.

Ch5 Strengthening

Standing Squat on Foam Roller

TARGET AREAS:

Buttock and leg muscles.

hold:
3 seconds

repeat:
1–3 set(s),
6–12 reps

frequency:
2–3 times per week

notes

BENEFITS:

Performing a standing squat on a roller will improve your body mechanics when lifting boxes or heavy objects from the floor or in and out of your car. This exercise will also improve your balance and strengthen your legs and buttocks.

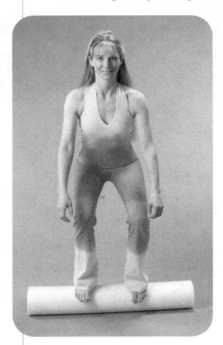

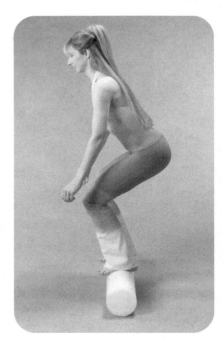

INSTRUCTION:

Stand on roller with feet hip-width apart. Bend knees and raise arms out in front of body as necessary for balance. Maintain a neutral neck and spine (a position where back and neck are not arched or flat, they are somewhere in between). Return to standing position.

Ch5 Strengthening

Standing Squat with Second Roller ★★★★☆

VARIATION:

Performing a standing squat with a roller in front of your body helps counter balance the weight shift posteriorly (backward). Standing on a foam roller will improve your balance and strengthen your legs and buttocks.

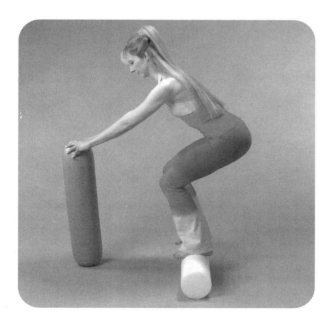

INSTRUCTION:

Stand on roller with feet hip-width apart. Position second roller vertically in front of body and place hands on top of roller. Bend knees. Maintain a neutral neck and spine (a position where back and neck are not arched or flat, they are somewhere in between). Return to standing position.

ROLLERS...

| ✓ | FOAM |
| X✓ | INFLATABLE |

Stand only on a foam roller, however an inflatable or foam roller can be used in the vertical positon.

TARGET AREAS:
Buttock and leg muscles.

hold:
3 seconds

repeat:
1–3 set(s), 6–12 reps

frequency:
3 times per week

- Keep knees aligned over feet while squatting.
- Standing on a half roller is typically easier than standing on a full roller as depicted.

★★★★☆

Standing Skater

ROLLERS...

✓ FOAM

✓ INFLATABLE

TARGET AREAS:

Abdomen, back, buttock, and leg muscles.

hold:
3-5 seconds

repeat:
1-2 set(s)
3-8 reps each side

frequency:
2-3 times per week

HELPFUL HINTS:

■ Keep knees aligned over feet.

■ Neutral neck and spine: A position where back and neck are not arched or flat, but somewhere in between.

BENEFITS:

The Standing Skater improves knee stability and increases strength in the core, and upper and lower body.

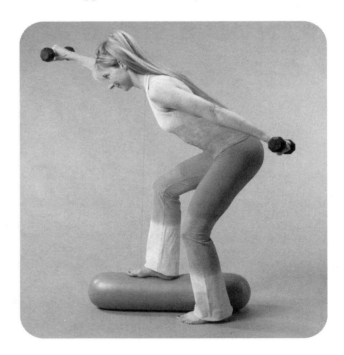

INSTRUCTION:

Holding dumbbells, stand with right foot positioned slightly in front of left on top as show above. Gently draw lower abdomen toward spine. Lean forward at waist, bend knees slightly, and raise right arm to ear height and extend left arm to hip height. Maintain a neutral neck and spine. Hold. Return to standing position. Perform exercise on opposite leg.

Flow Chart

Exercise:	Set	Date	Hold Time	sets 1	sets 2	sets 3	Exercise Heart Rate	Date	Hold Time	sets 1	sets 2	sets 3	Exercise Heart Rate	Date	Hold Time	sets 1	sets 2	sets 3	Exercise Heart Rate
Standing Skater *(example)*	Reps	1/1	3	5	5		125	1/4	4	5	5		120	1/8	5	6	6		110
	Reps																		
	Reps																		
	Reps																		
	Reps																		
	Reps																		
	Reps																		
	Reps																		
	Reps																		
	Reps																		
	Reps																		
	Reps																		

Core Strength Training   **Ch5 Strengthening**

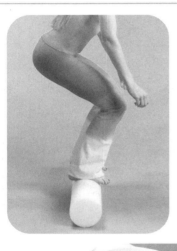
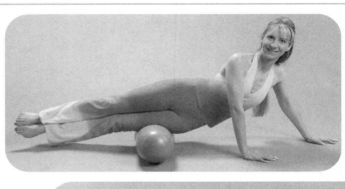

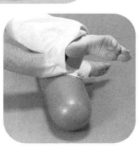
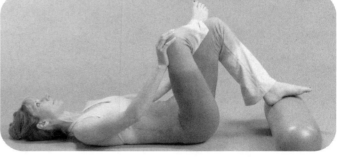

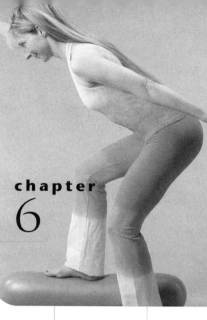

Mini-Workouts

The mini-workouts are designed as a quick reference to the exercises illustrated throughout the book, and to give you workout routine ideas. Perform these routines only after reading this entire book and understanding the exercises.

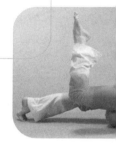

I designed the *Core Strength Training* mini-workouts to provide time-efficient workouts that can be squeezed into any part of your day. Each workout takes 10 minutes, or less, to perform. These mini-workouts may be used one at a time or several at a time to make a 20 or 30-minute workout.

Each of the mini-workouts has been rated on a one to five star system. One star signifies the most basic exercise level, two stars—advanced beginner, three stars—intermediate, four stars—advanced, and five stars—expert. The star rating is located at the top of the page. If the workout received one star, then you will know right away that this workout may be performed by a beginner, and a five star workout means you may need to wait awhile before you perform this routine, or that this routine is for you if you are already in great shape.

Once you have mastered all the one star workouts, progress to two star workouts. Progress to the next level of difficulty only after perfecting your current workout level. Keep in mind, it is more difficult to perform a workout routine than it is to perform individual exercises. Five, one star exercises performed consecutively is much more difficult than performing a single one star exercise.

These mini-workouts may be used one at a time or several at a time to make a 20 or 30-minute workout.

All of the mini-workouts have a recommended frequency, number of repetitions and sets, rest break, and hold times. This serves as a guideline, and ultimately, you must decide how many repetitions, sets, frequencies, etc., are best for you by following the established guidelines in this book.

I hope you enjoy these fun, time and energy-efficient workouts. The mini-workout pages are designed to be torn out, so you can post them on a wall, or take them with you.

—Caroline Corning Creager

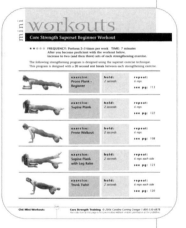

6.1 Mini-workout Page

Mini-Workouts

mini workouts

The 5 Essential Core Exercises

★ ★ ☆ ☆ ☆   **FREQUENCY:** Perform 1 – 3 times per day or as tolerated   **TIME:** 10 minutes

Master this exercise regimen before progressing on to ★★★ to ★★★★★ mini-workouts.
Rest 30 seconds between exercises or as needed.

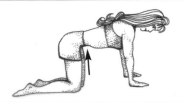	**exercise:** Neck Stabilizer	**hold:** *10 seconds*	**repeat:** *10 reps* **see pg:** *24*
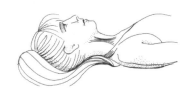	**exercise:** Scapular Stabilizer	**hold:** *10 seconds*	**repeat:** *10 reps* **see pg:** *25*
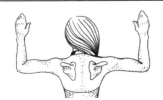	**exercise:** Transverse Abdominis Raise	**hold:** *10 seconds*	**repeat:** *10 reps* **see pg:** *26*
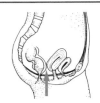	**exercise:** Kegel	**hold:** *10 seconds*	**repeat:** *10 reps* **see pg:** *27*
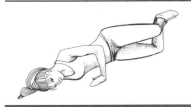	**exercise:** Hip Stabilizer	**hold:** *3 seconds*	**repeat:** *10 reps each side* **see pg:** *28*

Core Strength Training *© 2006 Caroline Corning Creager 1-800-530-6878*

workouts

Upper and Mid-Back Stretches

FREQUENCY: Perform 1 time per day or as needed   TIME: 5 minutes   ★ ☆ ☆ ☆ ☆

The following stretching program can be used before or after an aerobic or core strengthening workout, or any time throughout the day. This exercise program is designed **without a rest break** between stretches.

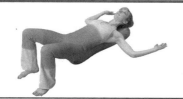

exercise: Chest Stretch	**hold:** 20 seconds	**repeat:** 2–3 reps **see pg:** 34

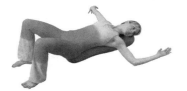

exercise: Axillary Stretch	**hold:** 20 seconds	**repeat:** 2–3 reps **see pg:** 35

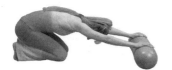

exercise: Shoulder Stretch	**hold:** 20 seconds	**repeat:** 2–3 reps **see pg:** 36

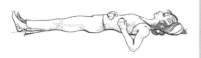

exercise: Diaphragmatic Breathing	**hold:** *inhale 3 seconds* *exhale 3 seconds*	**repeat:** 20 seconds **see pg:** 29

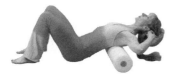

exercise: Mid-Back Stretch	**hold:** 20 seconds	**repeat:** 2–3 reps **see pg:** 38

169

Abdominal and Lower Back Stretches

★ ☆ ☆ ☆ ☆ **FREQUENCY: Perform 1 time per day or as needed** **TIME: 5 minutes**

The following stretching program can be used before or after an aerobic or core strengthening workout, or any time throughout the day. This exercise program is designed **without a rest break** between stretches.

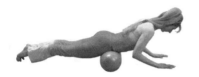	**exercise:** Low Back Stretch	**hold:** *20 seconds*	**repeat:** *2–3 reps* **see pg:** *39*
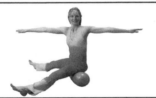	**exercise:** Trunk Rotation	**hold:** *20 seconds*	**repeat:** *2–3 reps* **see pg:** *43*
	exercise: Pelvic Tilts	**hold:** *20 seconds*	**repeat:** *2–3 reps* **see pg:** *40*
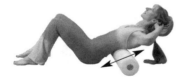	**exercise:** Back Massage	**hold:** *20 seconds*	**repeat:** *2–3 reps* **see pg:** *37*

Core Strength Training *© 2006 Caroline Corning Creager 1-800-530-6878*

workouts

Hip and Buttock Stretches

FREQUENCY: Perform 1 time per day or as needed   TIME: 7 minutes   ★★★★☆

The following stretching program can be used before or after an aerobic or core strengthening workout, or any time throughout the day. This exercise program is designed **without a rest break** between stretches.

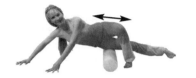

exercise:	hold:	repeat:
Iliotibial Band Massage	20 seconds	2–3 reps
		see pg: 44

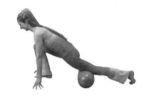

exercise:	hold:	repeat:
Hip Flexor Stretch	20 seconds	2–3 reps
		see pg: 48

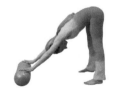

exercise:	hold:	repeat:
Downward Dog	20 seconds	2–3 reps
		see pg: 54

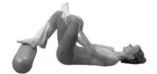

exercise:	hold:	repeat:
Piriformis Stretch	20 seconds	2–3 reps
		see pg: 46

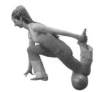

exercise:	hold:	repeat:
Hip Flexor and Quadriceps Stretch	20 seconds	2–3 reps
		see pg: 49

Ch6 Mini-Workouts

Lower Body Stretches

★ ★ ☆ ☆ ☆ **FREQUENCY: Perform 1 time per day or as needed   TIME: 7 minutes**

The following stretching program can be used before or after an aerobic or core strengthening workout, or any time throughout the day. This exercise program is designed **without a rest break** between stretches.

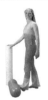

| **exercise:** Soleus Stretch | **hold:** 20 seconds | **repeat:** 2–3 reps

see pg: 53 |

| **exercise:** Calf Stretch | **hold:** 20 seconds | **repeat:** 2–3 reps

see pg: 52 |

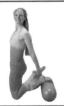

| **exercise:** Kneeling Quadriceps Stretch | **hold:** 20 seconds | **repeat:** 2–3 reps

see pg: 51 |

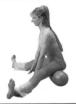

| **exercise:** Hamstring Stretch | **hold:** 20 seconds | **repeat:** 2–3 reps

see pg: 42 |

| **exercise:** Prone Quadriceps Stretch | **hold:** 20 seconds | **repeat:** 2–3 reps

see pg: 47 |

FREQUENCY: Perform 1 time per day   TIME: 10 minutes   ★ ☆ ☆ ☆ ☆

The following exercise program is wonderful for individuals who exhibit the rounded shoulders, and arched back look. This exercise program is designed **without a rest break** between exercises. After you become proficient with the workout below, increase to two (and then three) sets of each exercise.

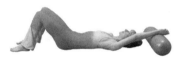

exercise:	**hold:**	**repeat:**
Chest Stretch	20 seconds	2–3 reps
		see pg: 34

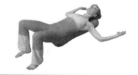

exercise:	**hold:**	**repeat:**
Lower Trapezius Press	3 seconds	10 reps each side
		see pg: 84

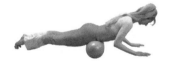

exercise:	**hold:**	**repeat:**
Low Back Stretch	20 seconds	2–3 reps
		see pg: 39

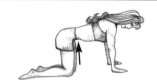

exercise:	**hold:**	**repeat:**
Transverse Abdominis Raise	15 seconds	10 reps
		see pg: 26

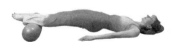

exercise:	**hold:**	**repeat:**
Straight Leg Hip Lift	3 seconds	10 reps
		see pg: 132

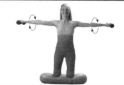

exercise:	**hold:**	**repeat:**
Shoulder Circles	1 seconds	10 reps clockwise & counter clockwise
		see pg: 76

173

Upper Body Superset

★ ★ ☆ ☆ **FREQUENCY:** Perform 2–3 times per week or as needed.   **TIME:** Varies
After you become proficient with the workout below,
increase to two (and then three) sets of each exercise.

The following strengthening program is designed using the superset exercise technique.
This exercise program is designed **without a rest break** between exercises.

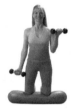

exercise:	**hold:**	**repeat:**
Unilateral Bicep Curl	2 seconds	10 reps each side **see pg:** 64

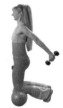

exercise:	**hold:**	**repeat:**
Unilateral Tricep Extension	2 seconds	10 reps each side **see pg:** 66

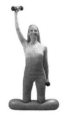

exercise:	**hold:**	**repeat:**
Unilateral Shoulder Flexion	2 seconds	10 reps each side **see pg:** 69

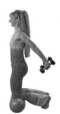

exercise:	**hold:**	**repeat:**
Bilateral Shoulder Extension	2 seconds	10 reps **see pg:** 72

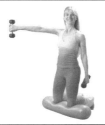

exercise:
Supraspinatus
Raise

hold:
2 seconds

repeat:
10 reps each side

see pg: *74*

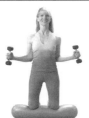

exercise:
Shoulder
External
Rotation

hold:
2 seconds

repeat:
10 reps

see pg: *75*

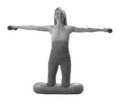

exercise:
Shoulder
Abduction

hold:
2 seconds

repeat:
10 reps

see pg: *77*

Ch6 Mini-Workouts

Upper Body Compound Workout

★ ★ ★ ☆ ☆ **FREQUENCY:** Perform 1 time per day • 2–3 times per week   **TIME: 7 minutes**
After you become proficient with the workout below,
increase to two (and then three) sets of each strengthening exercise.

The following strengthening program is designed using the compound exercise technique.
This program is designed with a **20 second rest break** between each strengthening exercise.

exercise:	hold:	repeat:
Tricep Press	2 seconds	10 reps each side
		see pg: 68

exercise:	hold:	repeat:
Bilateral Tricep Extension	2 seconds	10 reps
		see pg: 67

exercise:	hold:	repeat:
Bilateral Bicep Curl	2 seconds	10 reps
		see pg: 65

exercise:	hold:	repeat:
Push-Up on Roller–Beginner	2 seconds	10 reps
		see pg: 85

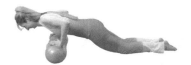

exercise:	hold:	repeat:
Lower Trapezius Press	3 seconds	10 reps each side
		see pg: 84

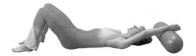

exercise:	hold:	repeat:
Supine Shoulder Half Pulses	1 second	10 reps each side
		see pg: 83

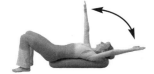

Ch6 Mini-Workouts   **Core Strength Training** © 2006 Caroline Corning Creager 1-800-530-6878

workouts

Upper Body Pre-exhaustion Workout

FREQUENCY: Perform 1 time per day • 2–3 times per week   **TIME:** 7 minutes ★ ★ ★ ☆
After you become proficient with the workout below,
increase to two (and then three) sets of each strengthening exercise.

The following strengthening program is designed using the pre-exhaust exercise technique.
This program is designed with a **20 second rest break** between each strengthening exercise.

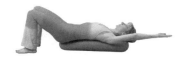

| **exercise:** Supine Shoulder Flexion/Extension | **hold:** 2 seconds | **repeat:** 10 reps each side **see pg:** 81 |

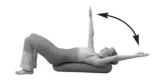

| **exercise:** Supine Shoulder Half Pulses | **hold:** 1 second | **repeat:** 10 reps each side **see pg:** 83 |

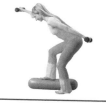

| **exercise:** Standing Skater | **hold:** 2 seconds | **repeat:** 10 reps each side **see pg:** 162 |

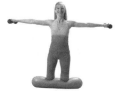

| **exercise:** Shoulder Abduction | **hold:** 2 seconds | **repeat:** 10 reps **see pg:** 77 |

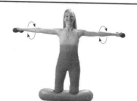

| **exercise:** Shoulder Circles | **hold:** 2 seconds | **repeat:** 10 reps clockwise & counter clockwise **see pg:** 76 |

Ch6 Mini-Workouts

workouts

Core Strength Superset Beginner Workout

★ ★ ☆ ☆ ☆　**FREQUENCY:** Perform 2–3 times per week　**TIME:** 7 minutes
After you become proficient with the workout below,
increase to two (and then three) sets of each strengthening exercise.

The following strengthening program is designed using the superset exercise technique.
This program is designed with a **20 second rest break** between each strengthening exercise.

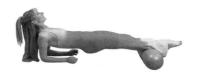

exercise:
Prone Plank –
Beginner

hold:
2 seconds

repeat:
6 reps

see pg: *113*

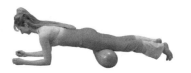

exercise:
Supine Plank

hold:
2 seconds

repeat:
6 reps

see pg: *122*

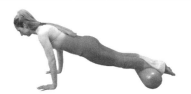

exercise:
Prone Walkout

hold:
2 seconds

repeat:
6 reps

see pg: *108*

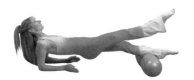

exercise:
Supine Plank
with Leg Raise

hold:
2 seconds

repeat:
6 reps each side

see pg: *123*

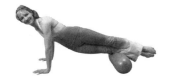

exercise:
Trunk Twist

hold:
2 seconds

repeat:
6 reps each side

see pg: *120*

---

workouts

Core Strength Superset Advanced Workout

FREQUENCY: Perform 1 time per day • 2–3 times per week   **TIME:** 7 minutes   ★ ★ ★ ★ ★
After you become proficient with the workout below,
increase to two (and then three) sets of each strengthening exercise.

The following strengthening program is designed using the superset exercise technique.
This program is designed with a **20 second rest break** between each strengthening exercise.

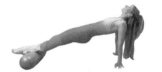

exercise:
Prone Plank –
Advanced

hold:
2 seconds

repeat:
6 reps
see pg: _114_

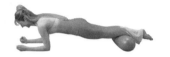

exercise:
Advanced
Supine Plank

hold:
2 seconds

repeat:
6 reps
see pg: _124_

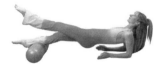

exercise:
Prone Plank
with Leg Raise

hold:
2 seconds

repeat:
6 reps each side
see pg: _115_

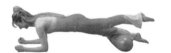

exercise:
Supine Plank
with Leg Raise

hold:
2 seconds

repeat:
6 reps each side
see pg: _123_

---

exercise:
Abdominal 'V'

hold:
2 seconds

repeat:
6 reps
see pg: _106_

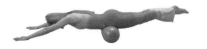

exercise:
Prone Tuck
to Swan Dive

hold:
2 seconds

repeat:
6 reps
see pg: _110_

Ch6 Mini-Workouts

workouts

Core Strength Beginner Compound Workout

★ ★ ★ ☆ ☆ **FREQUENCY:** Perform 1 time per day • 2–3 times per week   **TIME:** 10 minutes
**After you become proficient with the workout below,
increase to two (and then three) sets of each exercise.**

The following strengthening program is designed using the compound exercise technique.
This exercise program is designed **with a 20 minute rest break** between exercises.

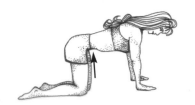

exercise:
Transverse
Abdominis Raise

hold:
10 seconds

repeat:
10 reps

see pg: *26*

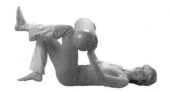

exercise:
Abdominal
Bracing

hold:
3 seconds

repeat:
10 reps each side

see pg: *92*

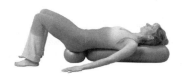

exercise:
Pelvic
Stabilization

hold:
5 seconds

repeat:
3 reps

see pg: *91*

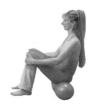

exercise:
Pelvic Tilt

hold:
2 seconds

repeat:
*10 reps forward
and backward*

see pg: *90*

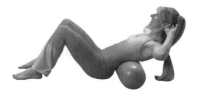

exercise:
Oblique
Crunch

hold:
2 seconds

repeat:
10 reps each side

see pg: *96*

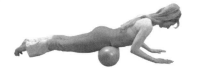

exercise:
Sideways
Crunch

hold:
2 seconds

repeat:
10 reps each side

see pg: *98*

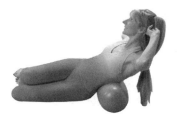

exercise:
Back Extension –
Beginner

hold:
3 seconds

repeat:
10 reps

see pg: *126*

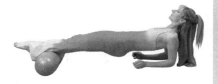

exercise:
Supine
Plank

hold:
3 seconds

repeat:
8 reps

see pg: *122*

Ch6 Mini-Workouts

workouts

Core Strength Advanced Compound Workout

★ ★ ★ ★ ☆ **FREQUENCY: Perform 1 time per day • 2–3 times per week   TIME: 10 minutes**
After you become proficient with the workout below,
increase to two (and then three) sets of each exercise.

The following strengthening program is designed using the compound exercise technique.
This exercise program is designed **with a 20 minute rest break** between exercises.

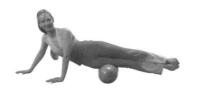

exercise:
Sideways
Tuck

hold:
2 seconds

repeat:
6 reps each side

see pg: 112

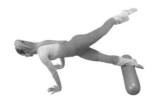

exercise:
Trunk
Scissor Twist

hold:
2 seconds

repeat:
6 reps each side

see pg: 118

---

exercise:
Back Extension –
Advanced

hold:
2 seconds

repeat:
6 reps
see pg: 127

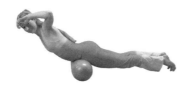

exercise:
Back Extension
with Rotation

hold:
2 seconds

repeat:
6 reps each side

see pg: 128

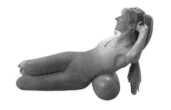

exercise:
Sideways
Crunch

hold:
2 seconds

repeat:
6 reps each side

see pg: 98

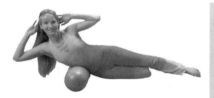

exercise:
Tummy
Trimmin' Trunk
Curl-Advanced

hold:
2 seconds

repeat:
6 reps each side

see pg: 101

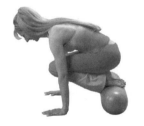

exercise:
Abdominal
Blaster

hold:
2 seconds

repeat:
6 reps
see pg: 104

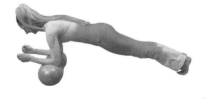

exercise:
Prone Plank
with Elbows
on Roller

hold:
2 seconds

repeat:
6 reps

see pg: 116

Ch6 Mini-Workouts

workouts

Core Strength Pre-exhaustion Beginner Workout

★ ★ ☆ ☆ ☆ **FREQUENCY:** Perform 1–3 times • 2–3 times per week **TIME:** 5 minutes
After you become proficient with the workout below,
increase to two (and then three sets) of each exercise.

The following strengthening program is designed using the pre-exhaust exercise technique.
This exercise program is designed with a **20 second rest break** between each exercise.

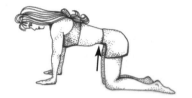

exercise:
Transverse
Abdominis Raise

hold:
10 seconds

repeat:
10 reps

see pg: *26*

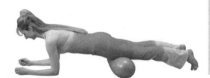

exercise:
Prone
Plank–Beginner

hold:
3 seconds

repeat:
6 reps

see pg: *113*

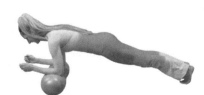

exercise:
Prone Plank with
Elbows on Roller

hold:
3 seconds

repeat:
6 reps

see pg: *116*

Core Strength Pre-exhaustion Intermediate Workout

FREQUENCY: Perform 1–3 times • 2–3 times per week **TIME:** 5 minutes ★ ★ ★ ☆ ☆
After you become proficient with the workout below,
increase to two (and then three sets) of each exercise.

The following strengthening program is designed using the pre-exhaust exercise technique.
This exercise program is designed with a **20 second rest break** between each exercise.

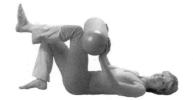

exercise:	**hold:**	**repeat:**
Abdominal Bracing	10 seconds	10 reps each side
		see pg: 92

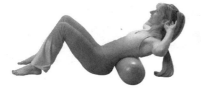

exercise:	**hold:**	**repeat:**
Abdominal Crunch	10 seconds	10 reps
		see pg: 94

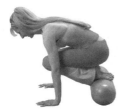

exercise:	**hold:**	**repeat:**
Abdominal Blaster	10 seconds	10 reps
		see pg: 104

mini workouts

Core Strength Pre-exhaustion Advanced Workout

★ ★ ★ ★ ☆   **FREQUENCY: Perform 1–3 times • 2–3 times per week   TIME: 5 minutes**
After you become proficient with the workout below,
increase to two (and then three sets) of each exercise.

The following strengthening program is designed using the pre-exhaust exercise technique.
This exercise program is designed with a **20 second rest break** between each exercise.

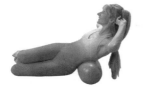

exercise:	**hold:**	**repeat:**
Sideways	2 seconds	10 reps each side
Crunch		**see pg:** 98

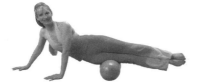

exercise:	**hold:**	**repeat:**
Sideways	2 seconds	6 reps each side
Tuck		**see pg:** 112

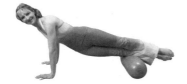

exercise:	**hold:**	**repeat:**
Trunk	2 seconds	6 reps each side
Twist		**see pg:** 120

---

workouts mini

FREQUENCY: Perform 2–3 times per week   **TIME:** 10 minutes   ★ ★ ★ ★ ☆
After you become proficient with the workout below,
increase to two (and then three sets) of each exercise.

The following workout program is designed to improve balance and strengthen the body.
This exercise program is designed **without a rest break** between exercises.

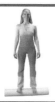

exercise:
Standing Position
on Foam Roller

hold:
1–3 minutes

repeat:
1 rep

see pg: *158*

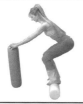

exercise:
Standing Squat
with Second
Foam Roller

hold:
2 seconds

repeat:
10 reps

see pg: *161*

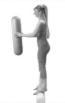

exercise:
Standing Shoulder
to Overhead Lift
with Roller

hold:
2 seconds

repeat:
10 reps each side

see pg: *159*

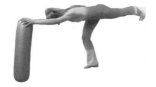

exercise:
Standing
Plank

hold:
2 seconds

repeat:
6 reps each side

see pg: *157*

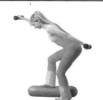

exercise:
Standing
Skater

hold:
2 seconds

repeat:
6 reps each side

see pg: *162*

Ch6 Mini-Workouts

workouts

Lower Body Superset Workout

★ ★ ☆ ☆ ☆ **FREQUENCY:** Perform 2–3 times per week **TIME:** 10 minutes
After you become proficient with the workout below,
increase to two (and then three) sets of each exercise.

The following strengthening program is designed using the superset exercise technique.
This exercise program is designed **without a rest break** between exercises.

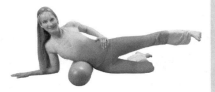

exercise:	**hold:**	**repeat:**
Outer	2 seconds	10 reps each side
Thigh Raise		**see pg:** 154

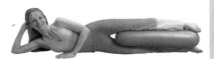

exercise:	**hold:**	**repeat:**
Inner Thigh	2 seconds	10 reps each side
Squeeze		**see pg:** 155

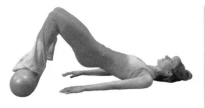

exercise:	**hold:**	**repeat:**
Hamstring	2 seconds	10 reps
Curl		**see pg:** 136

Core Strength Training © 2006 Caroline Corning Creager 1-800-530-6878

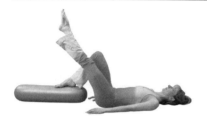

exercise: Straight Leg Raise	hold: 2 seconds	repeat: 10 reps each side
		see pg: 140

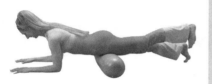

exercise: Hip Extension	hold: 2 seconds	repeat: 10 reps each side
		see pg: 148

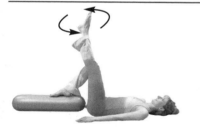

exercise: Leg Circle	hold: 2 seconds	repeat: 10 reps clockwise & counter clockwise on each side
		see pg: 142

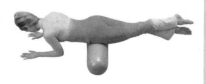

exercise: Criss Cross Heel Pulse	hold: 2 seconds	repeat: 10 reps over & under on each side
		see pg: 152

mini workouts

Lower Body Compound Workout

★ ★ ★ ★ ☆ FREQUENCY: Perform 1 time per day • 2–3 times per week   TIME: 10 minutes
After you become proficient with the workout below,
increase to two (and then three) sets of each exercise.

The following strengthening program is designed using the compound exercise technique.
This exercise program is designed **with a 20 minute rest break** between exercises.

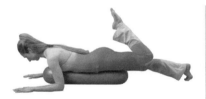

exercise:
Booty Buster
Leg Raise

hold:
2 seconds

repeat:
10 reps each side

see pg: *144*

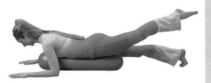

exercise:
Booty Buster
Knee Bend

hold:
2 seconds

repeat:
10 reps each side

see pg: *146*

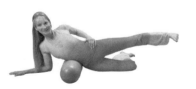

exercise:
Outer
Thigh Raise

hold:
2 seconds

repeat:
10 reps each side

see pg: *154*

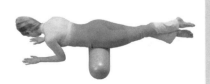

exercise:
Criss Cross
Heel Pulse

hold:
1 second

repeat:
10 reps each side

see pg: *152*

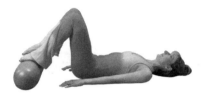

exercise:
Bent Knee
Hip Lift

hold:
2 seconds

repeat:
10 reps

see pg: *135*

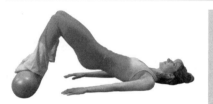

exercise:
Hamstring Curl

hold:
2 seconds

repeat:
10 reps

see pg: *136*

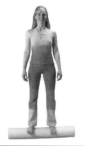

exercise:
Standing Squat
on Foam Roller

hold:
2 seconds

repeat:
10 reps

see pg: *158*

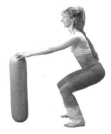

exercise:
Standing
Squat

hold:
2 seconds

repeat:
10 reps

see pg: *156*

Ch6 Mini-Workouts

workouts

Lower Body Pre-exhaustion Workout

★ ★ ★ ☆ ☆ **FREQUENCY: Perform 1 time per day • 2–3 times per week   TIME: 5 minutes**
After you become proficient with the workout below,
increase to two (and then three sets) of each exercise.

The following strengthening program is designed using the pre-exhaust exercise technique.
This exercise program is designed with a **20 second rest break** between each exercise.

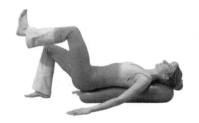

exercise:
Knee Raise
On Roller

hold:
3 seconds

repeat:
10 reps each side

see pg: *139*

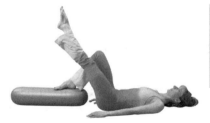

exercise:
Straight
Leg Raise

hold:
2 seconds

repeat:
10 reps each side

see pg: *140*

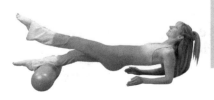

exercise:
Supine Plank
with Leg Raise

hold:
2 seconds

repeat:
6 reps each side

see pg: *123*

Core Strength Training *© 2006 Caroline Corning Creager 1-800-530-6878*

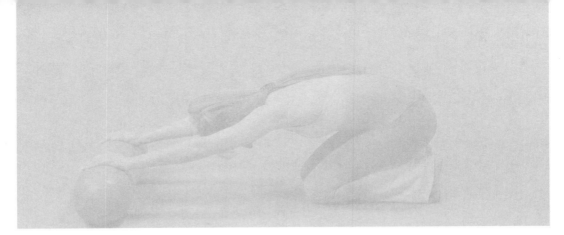

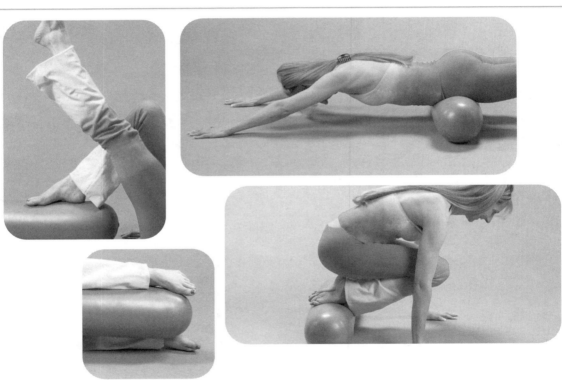

Aerobic Exercise and Physical Activity

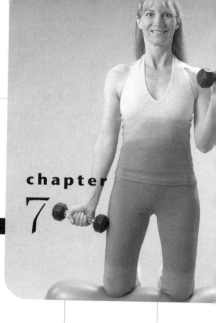

Aerobic exercise is exercise that strengthens your heart by maintaining your heart rate at a specific level above your resting heart rate, for a specific period of time.

The American College of Sports Medicine defines aerobic exercise as "any activity that uses large muscle groups, can be maintained continuously, and is rhythmic in nature."

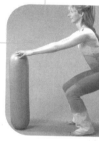

Performing the inflatable and foam roller strengthening and stretching exercises found in this book are wonderful, adding aerobic exercise, three to five times per week, in your regimen will further enhance your potential to burn fat, improve stamina, and strengthen your heart and lungs. Regular aerobic activity reduces your chances of heart disease and stroke, developing diabetes and high blood pressure, and helps build and maintain healthy joints, muscles, and bones. Furthermore, aerobic exercise promotes psychological well-being and reduces feelings of depression and anxiety.

The American College of Sports Medicine recommends the following guidelines when designing an aerobic exercise program:

Frequency: perform aerobic exercise 3 – 5 times per week.

Intensity: work your heart at 60 – 90% of your maximum heart rate.

Duration: exercise for 20 – 60 minutes.

Mode or Type: Any form of exercise that utilizes large muscles in a rhythmic manner, such as running, biking, bouncing on a ball, swimming, in-line skating, stair-stepping etc.

Alternate Activities Where Your Arms Can Swing Freely

Arm swinging, as with walking see (illustration 1.7), helps strengthen your abdominal muscles more rapidly. For instance, walk one day without walking your dog or pushing the baby jogger, and the next day go on a walk with your dog or the baby jogger.

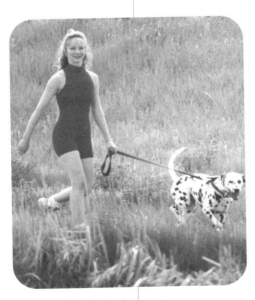

7.1 Alternate holding the leash in each hand to help promote reciprocal arm swinging.

When using a step machine, do not rest your hands on the bar in front of machine, gently swing arms back and forth as you step.

If you find that you are fatigued and overwhelmed trying to fit in aerobic workouts and meet the demands of your busy schedule, keep in mind that the Surgeon General's Report states that "physical activity need not be strenuous to achieve health benefits." You can select any aerobic exercise or activity listed below that you enjoy and are able to fit into your daily life.

Physical Activity and Health: A Report of the Surgeon General

"As the examples listed in the box show, a moderate amount of physical activity can be achieved in a variety of ways. Because [the] amount of activity is a function of duration, intensity, and frequency, the same amount of activity can be obtained in longer sessions of moderately intense activities (such as walking) as in shorter sessions of more strenuous activities (such as stair climbing)."

—*Physical Activity and Health: A Report of the Surgeon General,1996*

Examples of Moderate Amounts of Activity that Promote Well-Being

MORE VIGOROUS – LESS TIME

Stair climbing for 15 minutes
Shoveling snow for 15 minutes
Running 1.5 miles in 15 minutes (10 min/mile)
Jumping rope for 15 minutes
Bicycling 4 miles in 15 minutes
Basketball (playing a game) for 15 – 20 minutes
Wheelchair basketball for 20 minutes
Swimming laps for 20 minutes
Water aerobics for 30 minutes
Walking 2 miles in 30 minutes (15 min/mile)
Raking leaves for 30 minutes
Pushing a stroller 1.5 miles in 30 minutes
Dancing fast (social) for 30 minutes
Bicycling 5 miles in 30 minutes
Basketball (shooting baskets) for 30 minutes
Walking 1.75 miles in 35 minutes (20 min/mile)
Wheeling self in wheelchair for 30 – 40 minutes
Gardening for 30 – 45 minutes
Playing touch football for 30 – 45 minutes
Playing volleyball for 45 minutes
Washing windows or floors for 45 – 60 minutes
Washing and waxing a car for 45 – 60 minutes

LESS VIGOROUS – MORE TIME

BENEFITS OF PHYSICAL ACTIVITY

■

Reduces the risk of dying from coronary heart disease and of developing high blood pressure, colon cancer, and diabetes.

■

Can help reduce blood pressure in some people with hypertension.

■

Helps maintain healthy bones, muscles, and joints.

■

Reduces symptoms of anxiety and depression and fosters improvements in mood and feelings of well-being.

■

Helps control weight, develop lean muscle, and reduce body fat.

Core Strength Training

Ch7 Aerobic Exercise

Target Heart Rate

At rest, your heart beats slower than when you are working out. A normal resting heart rate for an athlete may be as low as 40 to 60 beats per minute. For a moderate exerciser, the normal resting heart rate ranges from 60 to 100 beats per minute. During pregnancy, the heart beats faster and it may take four to six weeks after giving birth for your heart to return to a normal resting heart rate.

The best time to measure your resting heart rate is in the early morning, before you get out of bed and start your activities for the day. This gives you a nice excuse to stay in bed a few minutes longer!
(Refer to the section on "How to Take Your Pulse").

When you exercise, your heart beats faster to pump more blood to your working muscles. Since your heart is composed of muscle, your heart is increasingly exercised as your workout increases. With exercise, your heart muscle becomes toned, and doesn't have to beat as fast to pump the same volume of blood.

To find out if you are exercising at an intensity strong enough to benefit your heart, you will want to record your resting heart rate, and then calculate your Target Heart Rate.

Calculate Your Target Heart Rate

First, find your Maximum Heart Rate by subtracting your age from 220...

Maximum Heart Rate = 220 minus your age

Your Target Heart Rate should be 60% to 90% of your Maximum Heart Rate...

Lower limit of Target Heart Rate = .60 x Maximum Heart Rate
Upper limit of Target Heart Rate = .90 x Maximum Heart Rate

You will want to exercise with an intensity that places you within your Target Heart Rate Range.

Core Strength Training *© 2006 Caroline Corning Creager 1-800-530-6878*

Example for a 30 year old adult:

Maximum Heart Rate = 220 minus 30
Maximum Heart Rate = 190 beats per minute

Lower limit of Target Heart Rate = .60 x 190
Lower limit = 114 beats per minute

Upper limit of Target Heart Rate = .90 x 190
Upper limit = 171 beats per minute

Always check with your healthcare professional before beginning an aerobic exercise program.

To achieve desired results, a 30 year old man or woman would need to exercise at an intensity that would make the heart beat at least 114 beats per minute, but not to exceed 171 beats per minute.

How to Take Your Pulse

Measure your pulse on either the carotid artery (on your neck) illustration 7.2, or on your radial artery (on your wrist) illustration 7.3. Use your fingertips, not your thumbs. Your thumb has its own pulse, so you won't be able to get an accurate reading. Use your fingers to apply light fingertip pressure to the arteries. Anything heavier may restrict blood flow.

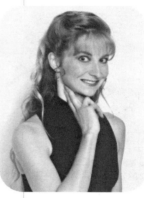

7.2 Carotid pulse.

Find your carotid pulse by placing the tips of your index fingers and middle fingers just below the jawbone on the side of your neck (top right photo).

Find your radial pulse by placing two fingers on the palm side of your wrist above the base of the thumb (bottom right photo).

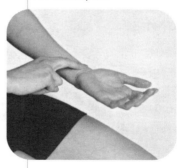

7.3 Radial pulse.

After you have found your pulse, count the beats for 10 seconds, counting the first beat as zero. For accuracy, use a stopwatch or a clock with a second hand, then multiply the number of beats you counted by six. This will give you your heart rate in beats per minute.

Number of pulse beats in 10 seconds x 6 = your heart rate in beats per minute.

Core Strength Training   **Ch7 Aerobic Exercise**

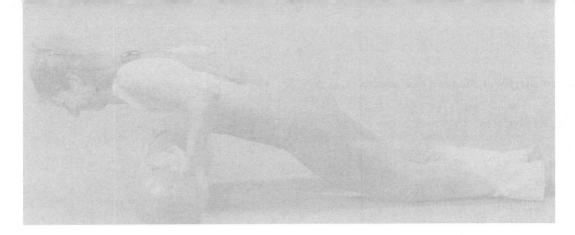

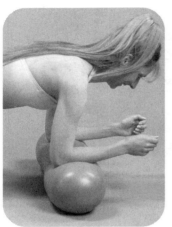

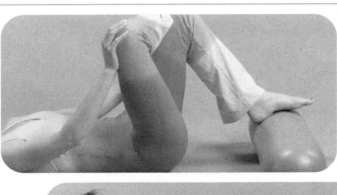

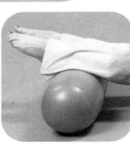

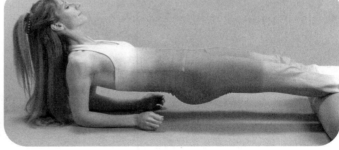

Core Strength Training *© 2006 Caroline Corning Creager 1-800-530-6878*

Glossary of Terms

Aerobic exercise: any activity that uses large muscle groups, can be
    maintained continuously, and is rhythmic in nature.

Bilateral: occurring on two sides.

Body mechanics: body positions used in activities of daily living
    to improve posture and lifting.

Bradycardia: an abnormally slow heart beat.

Carpal tunnel syndrome: pain or numbness in the wrist, hand, or
    arm, caused by swelling and/or repetitive movements.

Cervical: the neck.

Core muscles: the muscles that provide support and stability to your
    pelvis, spine, and abdomen.

Core stability: the ability of core muscles to control positional
    changes and return to their original position after being
    displaced.

Deep Muscles: those that lie below the surface; typically the
    stabilizing muscles.

Diaphragm: the largest and primary breathing muscle.

Diaphragmatic breathing: also known as belly breathing, is
    the correct form of breathing and is used during relaxation
    exercises.

Diastasis recti: separation of the rectus abdominis muscle in the
    midline of the abdomen.

Dynamic: the body in motion and its forces; opposite of static.

Exercise ball: a round vinyl ball used for aerobic, stretching, and
    strengthening exercises. Also known as a fitness ball or
    Swiss Ball.

Exhale: breathe out.

Core Strength Training   **Glossary**

External oblique muscle: mid-layer abdominal muscles, located on the sides of the abdomen, that assist with trunk rotation.

Exercise progression: a sequence of exercises.

Foam roller: a foam cylinder, or half-cylinder, used for stretching and strengthening exercises.

Friction massage: a massage technique used to break up scar tissue adhesions.

Iliopsoas: deep hip muscle located in the front of the pelvis. Responsible for lifting leg and controlling forward rotation of hip joint.

Iliotibial band: a sheath of tissue located on the side of the hip and thigh that has a tendency to become tight, especially in women and runners.

Incontinence: an involuntary loss or accidental leakage of urine or feces.

Inhale: breathe in.

Internal oblique muscles: mid-layer abdominal muscles, located on the sides of abdomen (beneath the external oblique), which assist with trunk rotation.

Inflatable roller: a cylindrical vinyl tube used for stretching and strengthening exercises. Also known as a FitBALL Roller® or an AirRoller®.

Intra-abdominal pressure: pressure change that occurs within the abdomen. When you inhale, the diaphragm muscle contracts and moves down, compressing the abdominal contents and increasing pressure on your bladder, bowel, and pelvic floor muscles.

Kegel: an exercise designed to strengthen your pelvic floor muscles, named after Dr. Arnold Kegel.

Lumbar: low back.

Latisimus dorsi: A wide, fan-shaped muscle located in the back.

Mini-workout: an exercise routine.

Mode of exercise: Any form of exercise that utilizes large muscles in a rhythmic manner, such as running, biking, swimming, in-line skating, etc.

Multifidus muscle: deep back muscles that work in unison with deep abdominal muscles to stabilize the spine.

Muscle substitution: using incorrect muscles to perform an exercise, as when fatigued.

Myofascial release: a form of manual therapy, designed to break up scar tissue adhesions between the muscle and fascia.

Myotactic reflex: a reflex contraction that is triggered by bouncing or sudden stretching of a muscle, also known as a stretch reflex.

Neutral spine: a position where back is not arched or flat, it is somewhere in between.

Obliques: abdominal muscles located at the side of the trunk.

Pelvic floor: muscles that support the pelvic organs, assist with sexual sensation, and sphincter control.

Piriformis: small muscle located in the buttock region.

Post-partum: after childbirth.

Pre-exhaustion: a technique used to focus on strengthening one muscle and follow it with an exercise that targets many muscles.

Prone: lying on the stomach with face downward.

Quick flick: an exercise designed to strengthen pelvic floor muscles and prevent urine leaking when coughing, sneezing, jumping, etc.

Rectus abdominis muscle: a long muscle located in the middle of the abdomen, aka the "six pack muscle". It often separates during pregnancy.

Repetitions: the number of times an exercise is repeated.

Rest: a brief rest period that allows your muscles time to recuperate for the next set or exercise.

Resistive exercise: a form of exercise that utilizes resistance, such as ball exercises or free-weights, to improve strength.

Rotator cuff: the four shoulder muscles.

Sacroiliac Joint: the point where the sacrum and the pelvic bone meet.

Scapulae: shoulder blades.

Scapular: the shoulder blade region.

Scar tissue adhesions: thickened scar tissue that occurs beneath the visible portion of the scar. May feel like a lump, and be sensitive to touch.

Set: a number of repetitions performed in sequence without stopping.

Static: stationary or at rest; opposite of dynamic.

Stretch reflex: a reflex contraction that is triggered by bouncing or sudden stretching of a muscle, also known as a myotactic reflex.

Superficial: muscles situated near the surface.

Supersetting: exercising two opposing body parts with a minimal rest break between exercises.

Supine: lying on the back with face upward.

Synergistic: an action, or coordinated movement, of two or more parts.

Tail bone: a small bone at the base of the spine, also known as the coccyx bone.

Target area: a specified area of the body identified for a purpose, such as weak abdominal muscles identified for strength training.

Target heart rate: an age specific heart rate that determines individual exercise intensity.

Thoracic: upper back.

Thoracic outlet syndrome: a condition caused by the compression of the nerves or vessels in the neck or armpit region, causing pain or numbness in the hands, arms, or neck.

Transverse abdominis muscle: deep corset-like abdominal muscles located on the side and front of abdomen.

Tricep: muscle located on the backside of the upper arm.

Unilateral: occurring on one side.

References

A.C.S.M. 1998. American College of Sports Medicine Position Stand: The Recommended Quantity and Quality of Exercise for Developing and Maintaining Cardiorespiratory and Muscular Fitness, and Flexibility in Healthy Adults. *Med Sci Sports Exerc* 30(6):975–91.

Baechle, T.R. 1994. *Essentials of Strength Training and Conditioning: National Strength and Conditioning Association.* Champaign, IL.

Bemelmans, B., Hankel, M., Jacobs, P., et. al. 1997. Pelvic Floor Reeducation and Body Posture Correction for Treatment of Female Urinary Incontinence: Results of Comprehensive Pre- and Post-Treatment Urodynamic Testing. *Neurourol Urodyn* 11:209–218.

Cosio-Lima, L., Reynolds, K., Winter, C., et. al. 2003. Effects of Physioball and Conventional Floor Exercises on Early Phase Adaptations in Back and Abdominal Core Stability and Balance in Women. *J Strength Cond Res* 17(4):721–725.

Creager, C.C. 2001. *Bounce Back Into Shape After Baby.* Berthoud, CO: FitNiche Publications.

Creager, C.C. 1994. *Caroline Creager's Airobic Ball Strengthening Workout.* Berthoud, CO: Executive Physical Therapy.

Creager, C.C. 1995. *Caroline Creager's Airobic Ball Stretching Workout*. Berthoud, CO: Executive Physical Therapy.

Creager, C.C. 2001. Foam Rollers Facilitate Core Stability. *WorldWideSpine & Industrial Rehabilitation* 1(1): 16–19.

Creager C.C. 1996. *Therapeutic Exercises Using Foam Rollers*. Berthoud, CO: Executive Physical Therapy.

Creager, C.C. 1994. *Therapeutic Exercises Using the Swiss Ball*. Berthoud, CO: Executive Physical Therapy.

Falla, D., Jull, G., and Hodges, P. 2004. Patients with Neck Pain Demonstrate Reduced Activity of the Deep Cervical Flexor Muscles During Performance of the Craniocervical Flexion Test. *Spine* 29(19):2108–14.

Ferber, R., Davis, I., and Williams, D. 2003. Gender Differences In Lower Extremity Mechanics During Running. *Clin Biomech* 18(4):350–357.

Hides J, et. al. 1994. Evidence of Lumbar Multifidus Muscle Wasting Ipsilateral to Symptoms in Patients with Acute/Subacute Low Back Pain." *Spine* (19)2:165–172.

Karst, G., and Willett, G. 2004. Effects of Specific Exercise Instructions on Abdominal Muscle Activity During Trunk Curl Exercises. *J Orthop Sports Phys Ther* 34(1):4–12.

Krivickas, L., and Feinber, J. 1996. Lower Extremity Injuries In College Athletes: Relation Between Ligamentous Laxity and Lower Extremity Muscle Tightness. *Arch Phys Med Rehabil* 77(11):1139–43.

Leetun, D., Ireland, M., Willson, J., et. al. 2004. Core Stability Measures as Risk Factors for Lower Extremity Injury in Athletes. *Med Sci Sports Exerc* 36(6):926–934.

Moseley, G., Hodges, P., and Gandevia, S. 2002. Deep and Superficial Fibers of the Lumbar Multifidus Muscle Are Differentially Active During Voluntary Arm Movements. *Spine* (27(2):E29–36.

Neumann, P., and Gill, V. 2002. Pelvic Floor and Abdominal Muscle Interaction: EMG Activity and Intra-abdominal Pressure. *Int Urogynecol J Pelvic Floor Dysfunct* 13(2): 125–132.

Richardson, C., and Jull, G. 1995. Muscle Control – Pain Control: What Exercises Would You Prescribe? *Man Ther* 1: 2–10.

Richardson, C., Jull, G., Hodges, P., and Hides, J. 1999. *Therapeutic Exercise for Spinal Segmental Stabilization in Low Back Pain: Scientific Basis and Clinical Approach.* London: Churchill Livingstone.

Richardson, C., Hodges, P., and Hides, J. 2004. *Therapeutic Exercise for Lumbopelvic Stabilization: A Motor Control Approach for the Treatment and Prevention of Low Back Pain.* London: Churchill Livingstone.

Richardson, C., Snijders, C., Hides, J., et.al. 2002. The Relation Between the Transversus Abdominis Muscles, Sacroiliac Joint Mechanics, and Low Back Pain. *Spine* (27)4:399–405.

Sahrmann, S.A. 2002. *Diagnosis and Treatment of Movement Impairment Syndromes.* St. Louis, MO: Mosby.

Sapsford, R. 2004. Rehabilitation of Pelvic Floor Muscles Utilizing Trunk Stabilization. *Man Ther* 9(1):3–12.

Sapsford, R., et. al. 2001. Co-activation of the Abdominal and Pelvic Floor Muscles During Voluntary Exercises. *Neurourol and Urodyn* 20:31–42.

Smith, C. 1994. The Warm-up Procedure: To Stretch or Not to Stretch. A Brief Review. *J Ortho Sports Phys Ther* 19(1):12–17.

Stanton, R., Reaburn, P., and Humphries, B. 2004. The Effect of Short-term Swiss Ball Training on Core Stability and Running Economy. *J Strength Cond Res* 18(3):522–528.

United States Department of Health and Human Services. 1996. *Physical Activity and Health: A Report of the Surgeon General.* Atlanta, GA: US Department of Health and Human Services, Centers for Disease Control and Prevention, National Center for Chronic Disease Prevention and Health Promotion.

Webster's New World Dictionary: Second College Edition. 1982. New York, Simon and Schuster.

Recommended Reading

Recommended Reading by Caroline C. Creager

Bounce Back Into Shape After Baby by
Caroline Corning Creager, © 2001; 198 pp.
paperback; ISBN 0-9641153-5-2

Caroline Creager's Airobic Ball Strengthening Workout
by Caroline Corning Creager, © 1994; 64 pp.
paperback; ISBN 0-9641153-1-X.

Caroline Creager's Airobic Ball Stretching Workout
by Caroline Corning Creager, © 1995; 64 pp.
paperback; ISBN 0-9641153-2-8.

Therapeutic Exercises Using Foam Rollers
by Caroline Corning Creager, © 1996; 236 pp.
otabind paperback; ISBN 0-9641153-3-6.

Therapeutic Exercises Using Resistive Bands
by Caroline Corning Creager, © 1998; 366 pp.
otabind paperback; ISBN 0-9641153-4-4.

Therapeutic Exercises Using the Swiss Ball
by Caroline Corning Creager, © 1994;
otabind paperback; ISBN 0-9641153-0-1.

Ordering Information

To order Caroline Corning Creager's books, exercise balls, or foam rollers, please call one of the following distributors:

Australia

Healthtrek: 1300 888 286

www.healthtrek.net

Star Systems: 07 3630 1696

www.starsystems.com.au

New Zealand

Product Zone: 0800 776 396

www.productzone.co.nz

South Africa

THERA-MED: 27 11 8046746

home.global.co.za/~dhtgo/

United Kingdom

Mastermedica Limited: 01684 311 444

www.bodycraft.co.uk

Osteopathic Supplies Limited: 01432 263939

www.o-s-l.com

Physical Company Ltd.: 01494 769 222

www.physicalcompany.co.uk

United States/Canada

Orthopedic Physical Therapy Products: (800)367- 7393

www.optp.com

Index

A

aerobic exercise 195–197
Agency for Health Care Policy and Research 20
American College of Sports Medicine 2, 57, 59, 195
arm swinging 196

B

back pain 17
Baechle, T. R. 58–59, 61
ball, small 80, 91
Bemelmans, B. 18
biceps muscles 64, 65

C

calf muscles 52, 53
cervical muscles 24
compound setting 60–61
core muscles
    diaphragm 16, 29
    exhaling 16
    5 Essential Core Strengthening Exercises 3, 22–29, 168
    hips 21, 28
    importance 1
    internal and external obliques 19
    intra-abdominal pressure 16
    Kegel exercises 20–21, 27
    locations 15–16
    lower and upper 21
    multifidus 17
    neck 22, 24
    pelvic floor 20–21
    rectus abdominis 20, 92–94
    scapular muscles 22, 25
    spinal stabilization 17
    transverse abdominis 17–19, 26

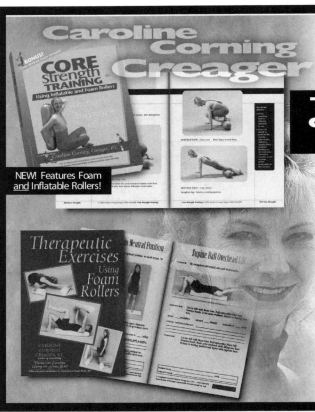
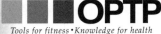
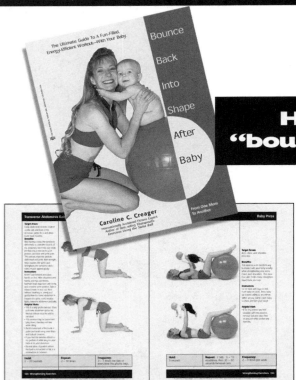